WRITINGS ON THE SOBER LIFE
The Art and Grace of Living Long

Alvise Cornaro

WRITINGS ON THE SOBER LIFE

The Art and Grace of Living Long

Edited and translated, with additional notes
by Hiroko Fudemoto

Foreword by Greg Critser

Introduction and Essay by Marisa Milani

UNIVERSITY OF TORONTO PRESS
Toronto Buffalo London

ISBN 978-1-4426-4509-7

The Lorenzo Da Ponte Italian Library

Library and Archives Canada Cataloguing in Publication

Cornaro, Luigi, 1475–1566 [Discorsi della vita sobria. English] Writings on
the sober life : the art and grace of living long / Alvise Cornaro ; edited
and translated by Hiroko Fudemoto ; foreword by Greg Critser ;
introduction and essay by Marisa Milani.

(Lorenzo Da Ponte Italian Library) Translation of: Discorsi della vita sobria. Includes
bibliographical references and index.
ISBN 978-1-4426-4509-7 (bound)

1. Health – Early works to 1800.   2. Longevity – Early works to 1800.
I. Fudemoto, Hiroko, editor, translator   II. Critser, Greg,
writer of added commentary   III. Milani, Marisa writer of added
commentary   IV. Title.   V. Title: Discorsi della vita sobria. English.   VI. Series:
Lorenzo Da Ponte Italian Library series

RA775.C6713 2014   613   C2013-908700-1

Publication of this book has been assisted by the Istituto Italiano di Cultura,
Toronto.

This book has been published under the aegis and with financial assistance of:
Fondazione Cassamarca, Treviso; the National Italian-American Foundation;
Ministero degli Affari Esteri, Direzione Generale per la Promozione e la Cooperazione
Culturale; Ministero per i Beni e le Attività Culturali, Direzione Generale per i
Beni Librari e gli Istituti Culturali, Servizio per la promozione del libro
e della lettura.

University of Toronto Press acknowledges the financial assistance to its publishing
program of the Canada Council for the Arts and the Ontario Arts Council.

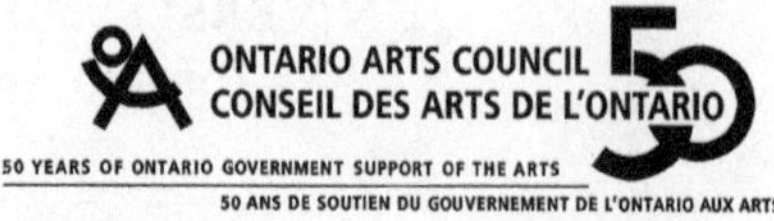

University of Toronto Press acknowledges the financial support for its publishing
activities of the Government of Canada through the Book Publishing industry
Development Program (BPIDP).

Contents

Foreword

If one were asked to name a telling aspect of the early twenty-first century, one would be hard pressed to come up with something better than the subject of aging. For the first time in history, elderly populations are overtaking young populations in both numbers and influence. The phenomenon is global; its impact wide and deep.

Hence today's newfound interest in longevity or, rather, pro-longevity – the belief that one can beat traditional aging and live an extra-long healthy life. Like Cicero, who believed that we ought to "treat aging as we would a disease,"[1] the contemporary immortalist seeks the "end of aging as we know it."[2] Modern society, too, is pro-longevist to its core, driven by the twin forces of an aging population and the consumerist medical engine that services it. Anti-aging medicine now surpasses $50 billion a year in revenue. There are anti-aging medical societies and magazines and TV channels. Politicians pander to the elderly. Sophia Loren is on the cover of *Modern Maturity*.

Where did we get the idea that we can seriously retard or stop aging? The dream has lurked since Pythagoras, but the notion that human agency might extend maximum lifespan arrives only with the Italian Renaissance. This it did in the person of Alvise "Luigi" Cornaro, and in his famous treatise *La Vita Sobria*. The book in your hand features the first complete new English translation of that work in more than 200 years. It is a remarkable work, one that elegantly

---

1 Marcus Tullius Cicero, "On Old Age," in *Letters and Treatises of Cicero and Pliny* (New York: PF Collier and Son, 1909), p. 58.
2 Aubrey DeGrey, Interview with Greg Critser, 22 September 2007. See also Aubrey De-Grey, *Ending Aging* (New York, 2007).

deepens, fixes, and restores. It also preserves and explains Cornaro's eccentricities, while making them more approachable to the twenty-first-century mind. In this and its accompanying documents, some of them translated into English for the first time, we can inhabit the world of the original immortalist.

Who was he?

Early Life

On 17 July 1509 the great Venetian general Andrea Gritti and a troop of soldiers docked at the Porto Codalunga on the outer wall of Padua and commenced to retake the city from its imperial captors. "Marco! Marco!" he cried out as a call to rally. As a sign of good will, Gritti presented to the besieged inhabitants a number of staple goods, along with "3 cara [di] formento" – three carts full of wheat.[3] The exchange, recorded in Marin Sanudo's famed *Diarii*, was meant to document the signal military event of early-sixteenth-century life in the Veneto, but it also, at least retro-spectively, brings together two transformative trends: land reform and politico-economic entrepreneurship wielded by the men who planted that land, much of it, eventually, in carbohydrate-rich New World crops.[4]

Alvise Cornaro prospered by them all. Arguably, he was also, at one time or another, sickened by them.

Born in Venice in c.1484, Cornaro spent his early years pursuing a dream: to restore his family's presumed lost noble lineage.[5] Over and over, in pleading after pleading, he insisted that he descended from the same line as Doge Marco Cornaro. The young man told a mangled, un-believable story, something about an ancestor in Morea who had lost his connection to the old line family. Not surprisingly, the keepers of the Libro D'Oro repeatedly turned him down. In the highly bureaucratized Venice of the period, that meant one thing for a young man: limits – limits on one's future, limits on one's ability to live the good life.

Fortunately for Alvise, there were options. His mother, whose family had the real money in the Cornaro household, sent him to live with an uncle,

---

3 Sanudo, *I diarii di Marino Sanuto,* July 1509.

4 New World crops – rice and corn – figured heavily in Veneto agriculture during the period. The "3 carts of wheat" may have been corn, given the use of the same word – *formentum* – for the new crop. See James McCann, *Maize and Grace* (Cambridge, MA: Harvard University Press, 2005), pp. 63–77.

5 The best single account of Cornaro's early years is in Giuseppe Fiocco, *Alvise Cornaro: Il suo tempo e le sue opere* (Venice: N. Pozza, 1965), pp. 15–44, and in Marisa Milani.

"Barba" Angelieri, in Padua, about thirty miles inland from Venice. It was a fortuitous match. Barba Angelieri was the classic political entrepreneur, obtaining municipal, ecclesiastical, and academic posts to further his economic interests. Padua itself was in nearly continuous turmoil, having survived the League of Cambrae wars by constantly shifting allegiances between Maximillian's empire and the Serenissima. The result was a culture of experimentation and relative openness. And opportunity; with Venice shifting its empire away from sea and only land – the result of setbacks in Turkey and elsewhere – suddenly the fetid marshy lands around it became a prize. Venetians began an aggressive series of acquisitions. The lands that Barba Angelieri owned soared in value. All this the young Cornaro took in, a heady brew of enterprise and action, intellectual synthesis and guile. The lesson: one could transcend traditional boundaries.

He tried attending law school and got bored; his "choleric" nature, he later wrote, made him a bad candidate for a profession given to abstract reasoning and rigid theoretical rules. Instead, he began to frequent the arts world. As a youth, he had joined a Compagnia de la Calza, one of the period's informal theatre and arts troupes, many of which displayed a dangerous pro-Imperial tang. Now, he began to meet poets and playwrights and architects. He travelled to Rome to see the recently revealed treasures, classical art that would transform his later life.

Following the ways of Barba Angelieri, who left him several large parcels of land when he died, Cornaro became a deft player in the power game of early-sixteenth-century Veneto.[6] Another entry in Sanudo notes how Cornaro and a band of mounted hunters once rode through the piazza outside of St Mark's and deposited the era's equivalent of a gift basket – ten roe-deer, two wild boars, two stags – "tutto lui mandor a donar al reverendissimo cardinal Pisani, per haver il vescovado di Padua."[7] Pisani later made him financial administrator of the Paduan diocese.

---

6 For a discussion of land reclamation and Cornaro's influence, see Denis Cosgrove, *The Palladian Landscape* (University Park: Pennsylvania State University Press, 1993), pp. 161–4.

7 "In questa matina una cosa notanda, che per piazza di San marco atorno et per corte di palazzo fo portato da fachini una cazason fata a Fosson per Alvise Corner, sta a Padoa, videlicet 10 caprioli, 2 porchi ciangari, et do cervi grande, che fo bel veder." ["This morning there was a thing to be noted, that through piazza san Marco, both around and in the courtyard of the palace, porters carried game hunted in Fosson by Alvise Corner, who lives in Padua, that is to say 10 roe-deers, 2 boars, and 2 large stags, and it was a beautiful thing to behold."] Sanudo, *I diarii di Marino Sanuto*, 27 January 1519. See Linda Carrol's discussion of this in her *Young Charles V: 1500–1539* (New Orleans: University Press of the South, 2000), pp. 24–5.

Alvise also partied. And it was decadence – *crapula, lascivia,* and *troppo ceremonia* – that finally drove him to his intellectual destiny.

Diagnosis and Prescription

Not long after he married Veronica Agugia da Spilimbergo in 1517, Cornaro began to notice the toll his lifestyle was claiming on his body. He laid the changes to his perpetually hot and bothered "choleric" disposition; Galen had recently been republished, and his humouric theories of health laid purchase to much of the sixteenth century's reading class. But Cornaro got sicker. By the late 1510s or early 1520s, about the time of the birth of his only child, Chiara, he reported two important symptoms: a "perpetual thirst" and a bad reaction to simple sugars, from pastries to fruit.[8] The modern endocrinologist recognizes these signs immediately: Cornaro was an uncontrolled type two diabetic.[9] (He may well be history's first named diabetic, predating J.S. Bach by more than 150 years.) He also had gout and arthritis, both, like diabetes, highly inflammatory conditions. Cornaro's physician, unarmed with a blood glucose meter, deduced a grave prognosis: his patient likely had but a few months to live.

There was one possible treatment, he said, though nobody the doctor knew had ever done it successfully. It required a radical change in habit. As Cornaro tells the story in *La Vita Sobria,* "the doctors informed me that for my ills there was but one medicine, available whenever I would resolve to use it and to continue unwaveringly with its use. It was the life of sobriety and order."[10] This new regimen required Cornaro to consistently eat much smaller quantities of food and wine than was his custom. He had to push himself away from the table before he was satisfied. The reason, as Cornaro later explained it, was tied again to a Galenic concept: the notion that a human body possessed but a fixed amount of "radical moisture" for living, and that this humour was used up prematurely by gluttonous habits. Sceptically, Cornaro tried his doctor's prescription. Almost right away, he felt better. "[W]ithin a few days," he wrote, "I noticed that such a life was greatly beneficial to me, and by following it, within less than a year

---

8 Cornaro, *La Vita Sobria,* trans. Hiroko Fudemoto, *Sober* ..., p. 79.

9 A discussion of a "cryptic diabetes epidemic" during this period is in Jared Diamond, "The Double Puzzle of Diabetes," *Nature* 423 (5 June 2003): pp. 599–602.

10 Cornaro, *La Vita Sobria,* trans. Fudemoto, *Sober* ..., p. 79.

(though it may seem incredible to some) I had recovered from every one of my infirmities."[11]

He then decided to experiment. Much of this is detailed in the following translation by Hiroko Fudemoto, but a few salient points deserve note here. Cornaro first tried applying the new doctrine to the dietary dictum of his day – that what tasted good was what one ought to eat for good health. "I found it to be false," he wrote, "because to me a very sharp cold wine tasted good, so too melons and other fruits, raw salads, fish, pork, *tortas* ... legume soups, pasta and other similar foods that delighted me enormously and yet all were harmful to me. Thus ... I stayed away from those types of food." The next piece of wisdom may interest those twenty-first-century folk who seem to be constantly searching for the perfect food. It was this: Quantity was more important than quality. He became "accustomed to my appetite never being satisfied by either food or drink, so that I would rise from the table while still hungry and still thirsty, in keeping with the saying: not being sated with food is a study in health."[12] He gave himself over to a sober and regulated life.

What, and how much, did Cornaro eat? The core of his diet was bread, in the form of pane padovano, broth with egg and bread, meat, and wine. He averaged 12 ounces of hard food a day and 14 ounces of wine.[13] This comes to about 1,500–1,700 calories. Perhaps just as important, at least in terms of what we know about diabetes, and, perhaps, life extension, was the nutritional profile of the Cornaro diet. It was high protein, high nutrient, low calorie, high fiber, and low simple sugar, save for the wine.[14] At its core was a bread made in the Padua region, *pane padovano*, contemporary recipes note that it was made with a whole grain, rough flour, and lard – strangely a kind of Renaissance version of the low-glucose breads now proffered by today's medico-health food industry; the fat (today it likely comes from some form of plant oil) lowers the glycemic load that is so injurious to the diabetic body, while the whole grain slows its metabolism and any harmful spikes in insulin.

The second part of his core diet was *panatella,* a thin broth – in Cornaro's case likely made from the capon – with small amounts of pane

---

11 Ibid., p. 80.

12 Cornaro, *La Vita Sobria,* trans. Fudemoto, *Sober ...,* p. 81. However, in the example of the William Butler editions (1903, 1917), the word studio from the saying – "il non satiarsi di cibi è uno studio di sanità" – has been mistranslated as "science."

13 The gerontologist C.E. Finch notes that this count falls well below that of the Minnesota Starvation Study (1950), and that Cornaro's intake was likely closer to 1750. C.E. Finch to Greg Critser, personal communication, 25 May 2009.

14 See A. Cappati and M. Montanari, *Italian Cuisine: A Cultural History* (New York: Columbia University Press, 2003), p. 130.

padovano and, sometimes, an egg. There are other versions of *panatella,* which Fudemoto takes up in detail later.[15] Suffice it to say that in 1522 Gabriel Zerbe, author of *On the Care of the Aged,* held that *panatella* was more likely a pap – water, sugar, and bread or flour; others describe it as bread and wine, and still others milk and bread.[16] I maintain that Cornaro's *panatella* was simply a diminutive version of today's *panado*: broth, egg, and small bread. I maintain this because of Cornaro's own juxtaposition of terms – "egg and broth" following "*pane padovano,*" and the complete absence of either milk or wine in the ingredients of the hard food he ate. Small note: A high-sugar diet would have made his persistent thirst even worse.

Cornaro's physical reaction to the regimen, he claimed, was nothing short of miraculous; at one point he jubilantly declared himself "immortal." He could once again mount his horse unaided and go for long rides in the woods, hunting, fishing, and staking out new lands for reclamation. Many of his conclusions ran to moralizing or Galen-izing. Often he mixed the two in the way a modern New Age practitioner might: "It seemed to me all the more reason that, if the world conserves itself with order and our life is nothing but the harmony and order of the four elements in the body, then it is order itself that should conserve and maintain our life; and conversely it means that life is broken down by illness operating to the contrary, or is corrupted by death. Order more readily teaches discipline. Order renders the army victorious, and finally, order maintains the City, the Family, and the Kingdom itself."[17]

Like many a reformed wastrel, Cornaro found himself renewed and ready to pursue passions long subsumed to the daily struggle of becoming wealthy. He took up a vigorous intellectual case for changing the entire landscape of the terrafirma; he travelled to Rome to get ideas for his own homes. There were artists to succour, political refugees to harbour, intellectuals with whom to banter. Something of Cornaro's state of mind in all of this might be derived from a letter, translated by Fiocco. Although ostensibly written to call attention to his (oft-overstated) reclamation of marshland, it also functions as an apt metaphor for Cornaro's own midlife transformation:

---

15 Gabriel Zerbe, *Gerontocomia: On the Care of the Aged,* trans. L.R. Lind (Philadelphia: American Philosophical Society, 1988), p. 218.
16 Cornaro, *La Vita Sobria,* trans. Fudemoto, *Sober ...,* p. 114n62.
17 Ibid., p. 87.

"The laughing meadows full of sweet and varied flowers and suffused in smell; the laughing woodlands clothed again in bright young foliage; the laughing trees full of so many different and delicate fruits; the laughing vines which release the sweetest odors from their blossoms; the laughing waters bubbling from clearer springs than ever before, their greater volume making a stronger murmur. So many different birds sing here, attracted by the clear fresh air, above all others the never-ceasing nightingale whose song is accompanied by the sweet notes of the cricket, the father of song. Singing, laughing, jumping, dancing and playing, the shepherds watch their flocks grazing over such nourishing herbage that they will make the sweetest and creamiest milk, so that to feed themselves they will require no other bread in their diet. All this singing, laughing and music-making comes from the new life brought to the hills by the liberation of which I have spoken, which has brought them back to their original beauty, as they were when the divine Petrach decided to live and die among them."[18]

Transgression in the Garden

On 8 January 1535 a small but remarkable notation appears in Sartori's mind-numbing *Archivio di San Antonio*, the principal catalogue of the famed church that sits just across from Cornaro's home on Via Cesaroti in Padua.[19] In it, the author notes something that occurred that day in "casa di Alvise Cornaro": the architect Gianmaria Falconetto died. The architect's sons were there to divide up a number of their father's paintings. Cornaro, we are told, was outside of Padua that day, but his *fattore* – his factor – had taken possession of everything of Falconetto's, apparently until his patron returned.

The entry shows how close Cornaro had grown to his artistic fellows, many of whom lived in his palazzo for years, even decades.[20] Gianmaria Falconetto is a case in point. Cornaro met him in the early 1520s, when Falconetto was still struggling as a painter. (In this oeuvre, his most significant – and controversial – was his "Zodiac" in Mantova for the Gonzaga family.) He was also a political pariah, his family having born

---

18 Cosgrove, *The Palladian Landscape*, p. 163.

19 Sartori, *Archivio di San Antonio ck*, v. I, p. 187.

20 A fuller account of Cornaro's relationship with Falconetto – and a full translation of Cornaro's *I Trattati Sull' Architectura* – is in Fiocco, *Alvise Cornaro*, pp. 44–53. Along with Lovarini, Fiocco assigns to Cornaro the bulk of the credit for the Odeo.

the shield of Maxmillian during the Cambrae Wars. For two decades, Cornaro's home provided cover.

The pair forged an important bond. Cornaro, the incipient humanist, used his resources to remake Falconetto as an architect. In the early 1520s, the pair travelled to Rome to see the recently uncovered Baths of Titus and Nero's Golden Room, classical sites that had so inspired Raphael. The experience was profound. Arriving back in Padua, Cornaro commissioned Falconetto to design and build a loggia, or outdoor theatre, near his palazzo. The result – restored and on display in Padua today – was a remarkable work: spare and sober of façade, with proportions right out of classical Vitruvius. It was "the first true expression of the Roman Renaissance in Northern Italy." From this work, and the intellectuals that gathered in Cornaro's garden, neoclassical values were "sprayed all over the Veneto countryside, fertilizing all kinds of neo-classical enterprise."[21]

Besides Vitruvius, perhaps the most powerful classical work to influence Cornaro was *De re rustica* by Marcus Terentius Varro (116 BC–27 BC), the prolific scribe's manual on agriculture and rural life. The work was revived by the nascent Venetian printing industry in the late 1400s, and Cornaro had almost certainly read it by the 1520s.[22] *De re rustica* celebrated the restorative and creative powers of rural life for intellectuals. It prescribed the essentials of healthy housing – villas should be situated for maximum air circulation, sunlight, and views of the surrounding area. His work also inspired Cornaro's continuing obsession with making terrafirma marshland into productive grain and vegetable farms.

Nearly all forms of entrepreneurship are transgressive, and Cornaro's was no exception.[23] At its core was the reclamation, through both

---

21 Douglas Lewis, personal communication with Critser. For an elegant description of Cornaro's impact on Palladio – and the political refuge he provided to both young Andrea and Giangiorgio Trissino – see Douglas Lewis, "The Training of A. Palladio," in *Macmillan Encyclopedia of Architects*, ed. A. Placzet (New York: Free Press, 1980), pp. 349–53.

22 Perhaps most on point was Varro's commentary on the undesirability of marshlands: "Great risks are taken in farming unhealthy land. By the application of such knowledge we can alleviate such risks in the cases of unhealthy marshes, unfavorable orientations, and direction of wind if some outlay is made." Op cit. in Bertha Tilly, *Varro the Farmer* (London: University Tutorial Press, 1973), p. 44.

23 Nearly all of Cornaro's writings on this subject are in Fiocco, *Alvise Cornaro ...*, pp. 99–155. See also Cornaro's "Scritti idraulica," in Emilio Lippi, *Cornariana: Studi su Alvise Cornaro* (Padua: Editrice Antenore, 1983), Appendix II. For a discussion of the debate between Cornaro and Sabbadino, see Manfredo Tafuri, *Venice and the Renaissance*, trans. Jessica Levine (Cambridge, MA: MIT Press, 1995), pp. 140–61.

draining and then irrigation, of wetlands all around the Veneto, mainly along principal rivers. The winding Brenta, running south of Padua and eventually into the Venetian Lagoon, was one key site. Cornaro had improved much of his own land there, and pushed farmers in the region to do the same. Although recent scholarship questions the physical extent of his reclamation, few challenge Cornaro's role as the principal political propagandist of reclamation. This he accomplished through his own writings, *Trattato di Aquae*, endless letters to *Signoria* bureaucrats, and debates with Venice's chief bureaucratic protector, the Savi di Prottetori di bene inculti, the Ministry of Unclaimed Land.

Cornaro's way was not always welcome, especially in Venice. The reason lay in one simple geographical fact, one that forged the mentality of leaders in the Lion City. It was this: By draining the terrafirma into rivers and then building embankments along its shoreline, reclamation increased the amount of water entering the lagoon, bringing with it silt, fresh water (instigating undesirable new swamplands), and raised water levels. The balance between sea and city proper was already precarious. More water meant more trouble.[24] Venice hired its own propagandist, Cristoforo Sabbadino, to make its case; not surprisingly, he eventually prevailed. In 1541 Cornaro was ordered to cut several important embankments so that the Brenta river, when swelled, would flow back onto terrafirma farmland, often upending the progress he'd made towards reclamation.

There were transgressive cultural tendencies in this Varroian neo-rusticism as well, and in Cornaro's garden one man embodied them more than any other: the playwright Angelo Beolco, also known by his stage name, Ruzante.[25] He, too, was a political refugee from the League of Cambrae period. He'd first met Cornaro in the early 1520s while performing one of his profane, bawdy works in Asolo, the little hill town that once housed Cornaro's famed cousin aunt, Caterina Cornaro. Beolco's chief literary innovation was his use of regional dialect – *Pavano* – in plays that ridiculed both aristocratic and peasant culture. He did this ingeniously by putting the contempt of the aristocratic class in the mouths of the peasantry, often using country bumpkin profanity – *pota! cancaro!* – and tales of famine and war. Today, many playwrights, including Dario Fo, consider Beolco the forerunner of modern *commedia*.

---

24 Tafuri, *Venice and ...*, pp. 151–5. See also Milani's "Introduction," in *Sober ...*, p. 57.

25 A brilliant dissection of the politics of the period can be found in Linda Carroll, *Angelo Beolco (il Ruzante) La prima oratione*, (London: Modern Humanities Research, 2009), pp. 5–78.

Cornaro took to Beolco, probably for two reasons: one aesthetic and one practical. In setting himself up as the principal humanist patron in the Veneto, Cornaro needed "content," as we call entertainment today, and Ruzante was prolific, memorable, and in some circles even chic – chic in the way, say, Black Panthers were in 1960s San Francisco. It felt good to be satirized – if you underwrote the clown himself. (Beolco once even sniped at Cornaro.) Cornaro himself appeared personally – albeit briefly – on the Ruzantean stage. Beolco staged his farce *Dialogo facettissimo e ridiculissimo* at Cornaro's country lodge at Fosson, on the way to Ferrara.[26] The other reason for Cornaro's beneficence was pure profit. Beolco maintained strong personal and cultural ties to the peasantry, and hence became instrumental in Cornaro's schemes to buy marshland and abandoned farms. By the 1530s, he worked nearly full time for Cornaro as a land manager.

There was nothing particularly exploitative about this arrangement. The context was dramatic and complicated. All around the Veneto came a profound shifting of status rankings. There was also a rural famine (1527–1530), continuing warfare, in-migration (from Romans fleeing the city's sack in 1527), Venetian meddling, the regionally new disease malaria, and ever-lurking plague. Heresy bloomed. Luther had proclaimed his theses in 1520, and his message was already percolating through the artisan community so dear to Cornaro's heart. There is little wonder that Beolco lived in Cornaro's *casa* for long periods: The theatre-loggia that Falconetto built for Cornaro was a perfect – and safe – place from which to lampoon the hierarchy.

We can get a sense of Cornaro's salon just by considering the mix of its principal members. There was Cardinal Pietro Bembo, the passionate (in more ways than one) advocate of *toscano* as the principal Italian language of art; one can only imagine his conversations with Beolco. There was Sperone Speroni, rhetoretician, early feminist, and defender of the *lingua vulgare*. There was Piero Valeriano, just escaped from Rome, who authored *Hieroglyphica*, the first Renaissance book of symbology; much of it was, from a papal point of view, troublingly Egyptian in origin. Daniele Barbaro, the cleric-translator of Vitruvius, built one of Europe's first botanical gardens just down the street from Cornaro's

---

26 For an example of their economic relationship, see Linda Carrol, *Angelo Beolco il Ruzante* (Boston: Twayne, 1990), p. 27.

garden. Both Vasari and Aretino later stayed as his guests and commented on Cornaro's "hospitality."[27] The notoriously freethinking medical scholar Bernardino Tomitano put in frequent appearances. A huge presence arrived in the patron-architect pair of Giangiorgio Trissino and Andrea Palladio, who likely lived with Cornaro during two anxious years of political exile.[28] (The Palladio scholar Douglas Lewis believes that Cornaro may have been the single biggest influence forging the young Andrea's breakaway aesthetic.) There was the future Cardinal Cornelius Musso, then a "boy preacher" living in the St Anthony seminary across the street from Cornaro's residence.[29] (Musso was so flamboyant and demonstrative as a preacher that he was known to don the dress of a woman just to make a point in a sermon.) And, of course, there were Cornaro's interior decorators, if we may call them that, many in residence for years. These included Lambert Sustris, the great muralist of Flanders; the sculptor Tiziano Mineo; and the fresco master Gualtiero Padovano.[30]

What did all of these men conjure? Palladio, of course, exported Cornaro's aesthetics to the entire Veneto; today one can see them all up and down the Brenta River. But a more vivid example of this intellectual garden appears in Cornaro's own Loggia and Odeon, the latter structure completed after Falconetto's death and largely attributed to Cornaro himself. The Odeon's interior stands in complete contrast to its sober façade.[31] Its ceilings burst with a near-hallucinatory admixture of sensuality and antiquity. There are satyrs and unicorns and Galatean porpoises, Diana Polymastes and Pan, rustic landscapes and sea-tossed ships, giant seashells, and endless arboreal displays. The few references to Christianity – some medallion-shaped plasters around the central entry

---

27 Vasari's visit is noted in his 1558 *Lives of the Most Excellent Painters, Sculptors, and Architects*, from the 1550 first edition, pp. 442–3. Vasari is also credited with first reporting that Cornaro desired to be buried with Ruzante and Falconetto.

28 Douglas Lewis, personal communication with Critser, May 2007.

29 Corrie E. Norman, *Humanist Taste and Franciscan Values: Cornelio Musso and Catholic Preaching in Sixteenth Century Italy* (New York: Peter Lang, 1998), p. 77.

30 One possible – but not probable, given the mores of the period – female in the group was Tullia d'Aragona, who was in Venice and in active *dialogo* with Speroni in 1542. See Janet R. Smarr, "A Dialogue of Dialogues: Tullia d'Aragona and Sperone Speroni," *MLN* 113, no. 1 (1998): pp. 204–12.

31 For spectacular photos – but *not* the text – see Vittorio Sgarbi, *L'Odeo Cornaro* (Turin: Umberto Allemandi, 2005).

vault – seem almost afterthoughts. This was a party house where boundaries stretched and sometimes snapped.

Two signal events foreshadowed an end to the party: one personal, one Europe-wide.

The first was the death of Cornaro's beloved Angelo Beolco at age forty-eight.[32] He had not lived a sober life. Menegazzo contends that Cornaro's blaming of Beolco's lifestyle was a dodge to distract from the fact that he probably died from malaria caught while tending to Cornaro's swampy farmlands. Cornaro, notified of his friend's passing while staying in tiny Codevico to the south, was distraught enough to write to Speroni about it. (At the time Ruzante was preparing to stage Speroni's play, *Canace*, at Cornaro's loggia.) The letter prefigures Cornaro's next obsession: converting his fellows to his brand of dietary sobriety. The letter notes how unhappy he is seeing his friends die so young, "even more so after the death of our dearest Messer Ruzzante." Cornaro then goes missionary. Such unhappiness "would have killed me from extreme sorrow, if this could kill a man, and before my having reached the age of ninety. But it was not able, because order has made me immortal, and has seen to it that at the age of fifty-eight I look to be about thirty-five years old, and every day this order makes it possible for one who is ill to regain his health."[33]

The second dampening of this Renaissance salon came from the Vatican, in the form of the Council of Trent. (Which Douglas Lewis hilariously has dubbed "the greatest party-pooper of all time.") The Council represented the Church's first official response to the heresy swiftly spreading throughout Europe. Its censorious impact on Cornaro was palpable and proximate. The first orator of Trent (1545) was the now-middle-aged Cornelio Musso. (He was likely no longer dressing up as a woman.)[34] The Council quickly ordered the setup of a new Venetian Inquisition, one intended to quell the Lutheran infection spreading through the artisan class.

---

32 See Emilio Menegazzo, "Tre scritti di Alvise Cornaro," in *Colonna, Folegno, Ruzante e Cornaro*, ed. Emilio Menegazzo and Andrea Canova (Padua: Antenore, 2001), pp. 340–1.

33 Alvise Cornaro, *Letter to Speroni*, trans. Fudemoto, *Sober ...*, p. 155.

34 For a complete discussion of Veneto artisans and changing religious affiliation, see John Jeffries Martin, *Venice's Hidden Enemies* (Baltimore: Johns Hopkins, 2003), p. 110.

Newfound piety reigned. One could almost hear the ghost of Ruzante: *Cancaro!* Increasingly, Cornaro took to the pen and tablet. The convivial garden on Via Cesarotti fell silent.

The Transgressor as Pious Croesus

There was much to write about, both from personal and philosophical perspectives. Cornaro again took up the cause of land reclamation, now routinely overstating his accomplishments.[35] He scribbled much on the subject of "Holy Agriculture" in a *Trattato di agricultura.* In all of this activity rang one overarching theme: order, sobriety, and health. His own, he claimed, continued to flourish. Once, when he got in a severe accident, he recovered quickly. And he was still riding and hunting in the "laughing" countryside. There was a mistress – Petrinella – and perhaps a child, suggesting another kind of health. Even his voice, often the first thing to fade in *i vecchi,* remained strong.

From this activity emerged the tract now in your hands: the *Vita Sobria,* begun in 1552 and written in instalments. In it surges the author's growing piety. True, the Letter to Sperone, pre-Trent, contained its requisite share of piety. Now, the Venetian Inquisition in full burn, Cornaro steadily inclined to Our Lord – and one holy Catholic apostolic church. In the first page of the *Vita Sobria,* he attacked three huge cultural trends unfolding in "O wretched and unhappy Italy": adulation and its rituals; "living according to Lutheran belief"; and *crapula,* or sickness resulting from gluttony. "These three vices, or rather cruel monsters of human life," he wrote, "have reduced our times to deterring the integrity of civil life, the religion of the soul and the health of the body." Of these monsters, he said, "I resolved to address this last one." What about adulation and Lutheranism? "I am certain that soon enough some noble spirit will take up the burden of censuring and removing them from the world."[36]

What followed must have been familiar – perhaps too familiar – to Cornaro's entourage, who'd been hearing about it all in the garden for two decades now. Alvise the Munificent retailed his life before and after the regimen, the essentials of his diet and the transformative powers of a *vita sobria.* "My sensory capacities are all healthy and perfect. My intellect is as sharp and clear as ever, my judgment sound, my memory unwavering,

---

35 The text is lost.
36 Cornaro, *La Vita Sobria,* trans. Fudemoto, *Sober ...,* pp. 76 and 77.

my heart big, and my voice, which before tended to be lower, is stronger and has become melodious, and I am now obliged to sing my morning and evening prayers in a loud voice, whereas I once spoke them in a subdued and low one. And these are all real and certain indications and signs that my humours are good and cannot be consumed."[37]

As will many when approaching their maker, he also started to embellish the record. As Cornaro progressed through various versions and amendments to the original *Vita Sobria* – one in 1558, another in 1562, still another in 1565 – he continually reset his birth date so as to appear older. The obvious reason was to better make his case for the anti-aging properties of his diet. He was "immortal." You could be too. His fame spread. In 1562 Tintoretto painted his portrait.[38] Musso, Tomitano, and even Sperone published letters and commentary on Cornaro's tracts.

Cornaro died in 1566; his true age was eighty-three. We do not know the cause of death. There is an account, published widely, claiming that "The good old man … did not look upon the great transit with fear, but as though he were about to pass from one house to another … having closed his eyes, as though about to sleep, with a slight sigh he left us forever."[39] Yet there are possibilities that the death was not so easy. For years Cornaro had complained that, at the end of summer, he took ill, often with fever, weight loss (suggesting diarrhea), and a pain in the side. Cornaro blamed the wine – his milk of the aged. By summer's end, he believed, the wine had gone bad. He claimed that revival came only with the new wine in September. A simplified version might be that the elderly tend to do poorly during hot and humid summers, for which the Veneto is known.[40]

Given the vast and swift changes in the environment of the Veneto, we might posit something else: *plasmodium vivex,* the main vector of seasonal malaria. Throughout the sixteenth century, with irrigation growing, the disease had taken hold in the region. We may attribute this to the rising prevalence of rice farming, which requires a careful, controlled swamping of land for the best yield. It is an ecology that evolves over

---

37 Cornaro, *La Vita Sobria,* trans. Fudemoto, *Sober* ..., p. 126.

38 Musso and Tomitano both issued cover letters to the *Vita Sobria* upon its publication; Speroni's ironic gloss on the work in ibid., pp. 140–8.

39 The original source of this account is usually attributed to the Florentine scholar and historian on Cypress Antonio Maria Graziani (1532–1611). This passage from Graziani is from Bartolomeo Gamba, "A Eulogy Upon Louis Cornaro (1817)," in Willam Butler's edition (see footnote 47) of *The Art of Living Long,* p. 188.

40 Cornaro, *La Vita Sobria,* trans. Fudemoto, *Sober* ..., p. 119.

generations. In China one finds a consistent and conscious maintenance of riverine and canal marine life. So too the fish that eat mosquitos and mosquito larvae, malaria's chief vector. The new, first-generation rice growers of the Veneto likely did not have such expertise, and so mosquito populations exploded, carrying with them the malaria virus. Did Cornaro's reclaimed land, his "Holy Agriculture," claim the old man in the end? Despite modern DNA forensics, we may never know. His burial site is unknown.

Legacy

For a period of about two decades after his death, the *Vita Sobria* was either out of circulation or censored. In the late sixteenth century one of Cornaro's grandsons sponsored a new printing. It evoked swift interest by Italian scientists and medical men.[41] In the early seventeenth century, Bernardino Ramazzini, the father of occupational medicine, lauded Cornaro's emphasis on hygiene and maintaining order in one's personal environment.[42] The Flemish theologian Leonard Lessius translated the *Vita Sobria* into Latin, appending it to his own *Hygiasticon*, a manual of healthful living.[43] The Welsh poet George Herbert, a sickly man who cured his bouts of malarial fever by strictly controlling his diet, translated the *Vita Sobria* into English in 1633. The book enjoyed wide circulation in England, eventually packaged with essays on the subject by Addison, Bacon, and Temple. Later English versions largely followed Herbert's trail.

Americans broke that mould.[44] In the seventeenth century the Rev. Parson Weems published the book under a new title, *The Immortal Mentor*

---

41 See Bernardino Ramazzini, *Diseases of Workers*, trans. Wilmer Cave Wright (Chicago: University of Chicago Press, 1940), p. xxxiv, for a summary of Ramazzini's *Annotationes* (1713), his commentary on *La Vita Sobria*. The original is under Bernardino Ramazzini, *Annotationes in librum Ludovici Cornelii de vitae sobriae commodis* (Padua: Jo. Baptiste Conzatti, 1714), pp. 1–88.

42 Leonard Lessius, *De la sobriété: Conseils por vivre longtemps (1613)*, ed. Georges Vigarello (Grenoble: Editions Jerome Millon, 1991).

43 George Herbert, *Hygiasticon: Or, The Right Course of Preserving Life and Health Unto Extream Old Age: Together with Soundnesse and Integritie of the Senses, Judgement, and Memorie. Written in Latine by Leonardus Lessius, and Now Done Into English By Leonardus Lessius, Luigi Cornaro, George Herbert, Nicholas Ferrar, Ortensio Landi, Thomas Sheppard,* trans. George Herbert (Roger Daniel, University of Cambridge, 1634).

44 Lewis Cornaro, Dr. Franklin, and Dr. Scott, *The Immortal Mentor or Man's Unerring Guide to a Healthy, Wealthy & Happy Life*, ed. Parson Weems (Daniel Fenton: Mill-Hill, 1810 [original 1799?]).

or Man's Unerring Guide to a Healthy, Wealthy & Happy Life, by Lewis Cornaro.
It was a highly edited version that took great liberty with language. There
was also outright censoring, the most obvious (and predictable) being
Weems's deletion of Cornaro's anti-Lutheranism. It struck too close to
the postcolonial bone. Weems deleted the Addison, Bacon, Temple bun-
dle and added essays from Benjamin Franklin and a recommendation
of the book by George Washington. It apparently sold well enough to
go into several printings. Cornaro became an early-nineteenth-century
staple.[45] In the 1830s, the whole-grain propagandist Sylvestor Graham
restored the anti-Lutheranism but used the opportunity to repute Cornaro's "quantity over quality" theory; in 1842 John Burdell repackaged the
Herbert version with a new essay on Cornaro's life by Piero Maroncelli,
the exiled Italian patriot and friend of Lorenzo Da Ponte, for whom this
series is named.[46]

Two early-twentieth-century versions dominated the nation's reading
classes.[47] In 1903, the Milwaukee publisher William Butler issued an elegant, gilt-edged volume, again striking the anti-Lutheran sentiments and
again packing in Addison, Bacon, and Temple. Butler was apparently an
early master at getting celebrities to endorse books; an auctioneer's list
of his printing plates and various ephemera associated with the books
lists Thomas Edison and Henry Ford, both of them heroes to the nation's middle class – and Butler's intended audience.

Sometime during the early 1920s, the idiosyncratic but prolific Haldeman-
Julius Company, located in Girard, Kansas, launched perhaps the most
populist edition of the *Vita Sobria* ever.[48] The company published the book
under the title *How to Live One Hundred Years*, and, more important for the
masses, sold it in its "Ten Cent Pocket Series." The books, in back-pocket
size, came from the offices of E. Haldeman-Julius, a free-thinking Kansan
whose other titles included everything from Voltaire to debates on evolu-
tion, socialism, and women's rights. All during the Jazz Age and well into

---

45 Sylvester Graham, *Discourses on the Sober Life*, 1833.
46 Luigi Cornaro, *How to Live Long* (New York: John Burdell, 1842).
47 Louis Cornaro, Joseph Addison, Lord Bacon, Sir William Temple, *The Art of Living
    Long: A New and Improved English Translation* (Milwaukee, WI: William F. Butler, 1903).
    In 1918: "Inscribed, 'To Albert D. Lasker from your friend, Henry Ford, Feb. 11,
    1928.' Newspaper clipping laid – in which states that this book was given to Lasker by
    Ford; 8vo; 214 pages."
48 Lewis Cornaro, *How to Live One Hundred Years* (Girard, KS: Haldeman-Julius
    Company, 1918?).

the Depression this version, Luther and all, circulated through the country. There is now evidence that it shaped the thinking behind the single most important finding about life extension to this day: caloric restriction.

Clive McCay, the father of modern longevity science, came from humble origins.[49] A native of Indiana, McCay was orphaned early on, and by the time the tall, rangy youth was eighteen, he had worked as a farm hand, itinerant hay bailer, and animal handler. Health and animals held particular fascination. Early on, McCay once recalled, he read a tract about the subject of calories. He was never the same. His sister once recalled how the young McCay never let a family dinner go by without telling everyone how many calories were in the potatoes and gravy, let alone the meat. He trained in the veterinary sciences, but ended up studying nutrition, then a red-hot subject, first at Berkeley, then at Yale and Cornell. There he made a seminal observation: Rats that were given optimal nutrition but calorically restricted lived from 30 to 40 per cent longer than those that ate normally.

In reporting this, McCay became a crafty, modern communicator. Writing in the September 1934 issue of *Scientific Monthly*, McCay noted: "Earlier experiments in our laboratory and [at] Columbia have shown that the mean life of a male rat is between five and six hundred days: if the average man lives fifty to sixty years, about ten days in the life of a male rat equals a year in the life of a man. In the present experiment the mean length of life was 509 days for the normally-growing male rats, equivalent to a mean age of 51 years for man. The rats of the two retarded-growth groups have exceeded mean ages of 780 and 870 days, respectively, equivalent to 80 to 90 years for man."[50] Then, almost as an afterthought, he added: "These data indicate that the potential life span of an animal is unknown and may be far greater than we anticipated." The potential lifespan of an animal is unknown and may be far greater than expected. Again and again for nearly a decade, McCay returned to these words. Maximum lifespan – in human terms always thought to be

---

49 L. C. Bing, "Old Salvelinus fontinalis," *Perspectives in Biology and Medicine* 13, no. 4 (1979), excerpted in Jeanette B. McCay, *Clive McCay:Nutrition Pioneer* (Charlotte Harbor, FL: Tabby House, 1994), p. 142.

50 C. M. McCay and M. F. Crowell, "Prolonging the Life Span," *Scientific Monthly*, November 1934, pp. 405–14, cited in Bing, "Old Salvelinus fontinalis," p. 486. See also the original study, C. M. McCay, M. F. Crowell, and L. A. Maynard, "The Effect of Retarded Growth Upon the Length of Life Span and Upon the Ultimate Body Size," *Journal of Nutrition* 10, no. 1 (1935): 155–71.

somewhere around the Bible's 120 years – was not fixed. So what was the maximum lifespan? Why, by 1935 there were rats in his lab that had lived more than 1,300 days – everyone knew what that meant in human years.

Where did McCay get his research inclination? Clearly much of it derived from his early studies of brook trout populations, where he'd observed the same phenomenon.[51] But a study of his wife's memoirs and papers in his archives at Cornell reveals a steady fascination with the *Vita Sobria* and Cornaro, one that was begun at least as early as the 1930s. At the time, McCay hosted a weekly radio show for the Cornell community. Often he talked about what he was reading – sometimes in science, sometimes in philosophy. In at least one program, he plunged into historic tracts on longevity. One of his favourite recommendations was the *Vita Sobria*. In the early 1950s, he suggested it as reading for his students. This is not causal evidence, but it is suggestive of the philosophical milieu that surrounded McCay's seminal observations. Not to sate oneself is the science of health.

Today, those observations form the backbone of huge, billion-dollar efforts by some of the most sophisticated science and pharmaceutical enterprises in the world.[52] Researchers at Harvard have developed what is commonly known now as a "CR mimetic" – a pill that mimics the effects of caloric restriction. The compound, called resveratrol, is based on chemicals found in red wine. In experiments of feeding resveratrol to mice, the compound pushed maximum lifespan upwards by 30 per cent. There was one telling snag: resveratrol's lifespan-extending effects seemed to come only in mice fed high-fat diets, a protocol decision, experimenters claimed, that mirrored the diet of the average American. When mice eating a normal, healthy diet were given resveratrol, there

---

51 Clive McCay, "Current Reading List Concerning Problems of Aging," typed
    manuscript compiled June 1950, in Clive McCay papers, box 10, Cornell University.
52 The basis of modern CR mimetics is in J. Kubova and L. Guarente, "How Does Calorie
    Restriction Work?" *Genes and Development* 17 (2003) 313–21; S. Hekimi and L. Guarente,
    "Genetics and the Specificity of the Aging Process," *Science* 299 (2003): pp. 1351–4;
    S. J. Lin, E. Ford, M. Haigis, G. Liszt, and L. Guarente, "Calorie Restriction Extends Life
    Span by Lowering the Level of NADH," *Genes and Development* 18 (2004): pp. 12–16;
    M.C. Motta, N. Divecha, M. Lemieux, C. Kamel, D. Chen, W. Gu, Y. Bultsma, M. McBurney, and L. Guarente, "Mammalian SIRT1 Represses Forkhead Transcription Factors,"
    Cell 116 (2004): pp. 551–63; and F. Picard, M. Kurtev, N. Chung, A. Topark-Ngarmm,
    T. Senawong, R. Machado de Oliveira, M. Leid, M. McBurney, and L. Guarente, "SIRT1
    Regulates White Fat in Mice:A Mechanistic Link between Calorie Restriction and Aging,"
    Nature 429 (2004): 771–6 (published online June 2, 2004).

was no lifespan alteration. What did it mean? Does CR, the modern-day derivative of Cornarian wisdom, only work with unhealthy people, and if so, wouldn't it be better to simply get people to eat better?

As it turns out, there may indeed be a use for resveratrol and like compounds in humans: even mice that did not increase lifespan gained huge health benefits, from lower rates of heart disease and, instructively, diabetes, the scourge of modern life. The diabetes connection warrants note, particularly in light of Cornaro's experience. In experiments involving yeast, fruit flies, worms, and mice, glucose metabolism was closely connected to longevity. Today, many scientists view diabetes as a form of accelerated aging.[53] Preliminary experiments with human diabetics taking a resveratrol compound have been promising. Merck, the pharmaceutical giant, has invested $750 million. Its competitors will likely follow its lead.

Still, if we take away all the scientific data, longevity claims, and diet wisdom, does Cornaro deed the modern reader something of value? Perhaps. Consider the essentials of his world: a new abundance of simple carbohydrates (corn and rice), often planted as monoculture; new and puzzling forms of infection (malaria); chronic disease (diabetes and gout); globalization of resources (the New World); and destabilization of existing political states. Now consider his reaction: voluntary dietary restraint, constant self-education, a vigorous physical life, convivial humanism. Were one to study any of today's popular manuals on what has become known as "healthy aging," one would find the very same recipe.

With a little *parmigiano* on top, it almost makes aging look interesting.

– Greg Critser
Pasadena, 2013

---

53 S. Imai and W. Kiess, "Therapeutic Potential of SIRT1 and NAMPT-mediated NAD Biosynthesis in Type 2 Diabetes," *Frontiers of Bioscience* 14 (2009): 2983–95.

Note on the Translation

A decision was made to preserve the tone of these early modern texts, that is to say, to conserve their sixteenth-century "voice." This was done in the belief that it would be a reductive act to render certain terminology – especially those classical or philosophical – into a contemporary vocabulary. Words specific to Cornaro's lexicon – *crapula, prosperity,* or the classical phrase, "perturbations of the soul" – have therefore been respected and maintained. This allows for richer meanings to inform the text, which would be less likely with the use of, for example, disturbance in lieu of perturbation, or thriving instead of prosperity. Said another way, by maintaining these earlier terms, it also reduces a natural tendency to attribute a single (current) understanding to that word. This is especially true in the well-known case of *animo* (Latin, *animus,* from the Greek psuchē), which, in its fullest significance, is the soul – some would even say the "human soul" as opposed to the "immortal soul" (*anima*) – as that which holds perception, memory, reason, emotion, or sensation: "the soul is that by which we live, and feel, and first understand." As a term, it can be rendered (and debated) in a number of ways – spirit, heart, soul, nature, mind, intellect, character, courage, intent, and so forth – not to mention the colloquial expressions for steadfastness, excellence, daring, courage, or even enthusiasm, again, to name just a few. A tendency to translate *animo* literally as "mind" has not been followed here for these writings – the reason for which is clearly seen in the examples given previously and the additionl note found in the "Selected Terminology."

The word *crapula,* a signature term, if you will, of Cornaro, denotes the ill effect that results from the act of excessive drinking or eating, and though it may be remote to our daily conversation, it still appears in dictionaries (*OED,* for example), as are its derivations: crapulous, crapulent.

Some would argue that the concept of crapula is better served by a more current term. One suggestion is intemperance, but Cornaro himself forgoes adopting this word – even though it was in use at the time – which more concerns the tempering of the body's humours. Another possibility was gluttony, but it is a term that, being one of the seven cardinal sins, Cornaro himself uses (*gola*) in a specific context. Crapula, for Cornaro, best conveys what is needless, in excess, or that which in Galen is the superfluous.

The Italian term *complessione* is rendered as *complexion* rather than as constitution or temperament, which is also in keeping with a Cornaro lexicon, adopted in turn from the classical and Galenic "complexion theory" of the humours – and signifies the body's composition in balancing the humours and the elements. The reader will become familiarized with such terms and ascribe these other meanings to them as he or she reads on. In an effort to assist the reader in this, specification of selected terms is provided in the notes or in the "Selected Terminolgy."

Translations of Cornaro's writings: All translations were done by this translator, except where noted. Translation of the *Vita Sobria* is based on the critical edition, *Scritti sulla vita sobria: Elogio e Lettere,* "Prima edizione critica a cura di Marisa Milani" (1983), by Marisa Milani (1935–1997), who was a Professor of Letters at the Università di Padova in Italy. Other sources are indicated in the notes and bibliography. Included in the Da Ponte edition are Professor Milani's "Introduction" (1983) and accompanying notes, together with her essay and notes: "Come raggiungere l'immortalità vivendo cent'anni, ovvero La fortuna della *Vita Sobria* nel mondo anglosassone," (1980) – "How to Attain Immortality Living One Hundred Years, or The Fortune of the *Vita Sobria* in the Anglo-Saxon World" – both essays are rendered here for the first time in English.

Notes inserted by translator: All notes by Professor Milani to her "Introduction" and essay "Immortality ...," have been included in the translations. However, the reader is advised that in regard to the "Introduction," and to the "Immortality ...," essay, information or notes within square brackets and designated by a diamond (◊, ♦) or asterisk (*), were inserted by this translator.

Ficino in Latin or Italian: In regard to Ficino's *Tre vite ...*, Milani cites either Ficino's original Latin, or Fauno's Italian translation of it. Where Milani cites Fauno's Italian translation – whose wording differs from that of the Kaske-Clark English translation of Ficino – a new English rendering by this translator was done based directly on Fauno's Italian.

However, where Milani cites Ficino in Latin, the Kaske-Clark translation has been used.

Double square brackets [[ ]] or asterisks **: These have been used to replicate markings inserted by Prof Milani. Double square brackets so placed indicate censored passages deleted from the 1591 edition by Cornaro's grandson. Asterisks so placed indicate text that Milani took from the *princeps*.

Variations on spelling: Throughout the volume, Cornaro's Italian title is also seen with capital letters (*Trattato de la Vita Sobria,* or *Vita Sobria*), which are earlier forms of the same titles written today as *Trattato della vita sobria,* or the *Vita sobria.* Cornaro's name occasionally becomes Aluvise or Luigi, and his family name is also seen written as Corner, or Cornelii. These are evolved variations on their names. Angelo Beolco, famously known as Ruzante (in *pavano*), is written herein as Ruzzante (standard Italian), following the Milani edition.

Punctuation: Throughout, punctuation adheres for the most part to the Milani texts, and any change was to yield a clearer structure to the reader.

The selection of letters written to or by Cornaro – illustrating some of the important figures that Cornaro knew and their response to his writings – are drawn from the Milani edition and presented in the same order as they appear therein. The exceptions to this order are the two letters by Sperone Speroni to Cornaro: the first in opposition to sobriety, and the second in favour of it. Not included here is the "Nun's Letter," originally written in French by Cornaro's supposed great-niece (*Lettre d'une Religieuse de Padoue, Petite-Nièce de Louis Cornaro*). It has an unknown provenance and offers uncertain information; for example, the day of Cornaro's death is given as 26 April 1566, which contrasts with the letter by his grandson Giacomo Alvise, who writes that he was alive at the end of April. Though the "Nun's Letter" is not included here, in Prof Milani's "Introduction," a French source is cited (note 71), and in her essay "Immortality," an English one (note 19).

In this verbal dance that is the work of translation, the author quite naturally takes the lead. Any missteps are of course the sole responsibility of this translator ▪ HF

Acknowledgments

A sad and heartfelt thank you is sent forth to Ron Schoeffel (1936–2013), who will be deeply missed not only for his exuberant good nature and knowing intelligence, but above all for the generosity of his great spirit.

I would like to extend sincere thanks to the personnel at the University of Toronto Press (UTP) for the production of this edition, in particular to the discerning Anne Laughlin for her always agreeable help in making things work, as well as to UTP's (anonymous) readers for their invaluable comments. I also thank the essential Emily Johnston at Apex CoVantage and her team for their much appreciated contributions to improve this edition. I offer genuine thanks to the following professors for graciously sharing their knowledge: Michael J. B. Allen (UCLA), Luigi Ballerini, (UCLA, Da Ponte series co-editor), Remo Bodei (Università di Pisa), Roberto Fedi (Università per Stranieri di Perugia), Giulio Ferroni (Università di Roma), Gilberto Pizzamiglio (Università di Venezia), and Elissa Weaver (University of Chicago). *Un grazie sincero* "crosses the ocean" to Piermario Vescovo (Università di Venezia, "Ca' Foscari") for his critical help in decoding the *pavano* verses and to Ivano Paccagnella (Università di Padova) for his contribution on his late colleague Marisa Milani. And of course, I thank the amiable Massimo Ciavolella (UCLA, Da Ponte series co-editor) for his indispensable help with the Latin translations. Last, though never least, my warmest thanks travel north to Naomi in Ottawa – tulips in bloom – for her welcome offerings of good cheer.

WRITINGS ON THE SOBER LIFE

The Art and Grace of Living Long

Introduction to Cornaro[*]

Marisa Milani

Premise

"Trattato de la Vita Sobria" [treatise on the sober life] appeared in
November 1558, printed by Grazioso Percacino of Padua. Cornaro followed it up with three other works, which – collected and published
by his grandson in 1591 under the general title *Discorsi della Vita Sobria*
[discourses on the sober life] – became a worldwide success. The present work proposes the first complete and corrected edition of Cornaro's
texts, and a review of the history of their birth and their long and fortunate life.[**]

---

[*] [NB: A note or text within single square brackets indicated by a diamond = (◊, ♦), or
asterisk (*) was inserted by this translator. The essay and notes were translated from
the "Introduction" by Marisa Milani in *Scritti sulla vita sobria: Elogio e Lettere*, prima
edizione critica a cura di Marisa Milani (Venezia: Corbo e Fiore Editori, 1983), cited
herein as *Scritti ...* . The English title of this Da Ponte translation, *Writings on the Sober
Life: The Art and Grace of Living Long*, is cited herein as *Sober ...* .]

[**] [Commenting on her Italian edition, Milani writes:] "Intervention on the [Cornaro]
texts cited from early editions was limited to regulating the accents and to spell
out abbreviations in full. Transcription of the *pavano* texts was done according
to those prepared for the forthcoming publication, 'Lessico pavano.'" [Prof. Ivano
Paccagnella (Università di Padova), co-edited that edition with Milani, and later
assumed responsibility for it. See Ivano Paccagnella, *Vocabolario del pavano: XIV–XVII
secolo* (Padua: Editrice Esedra, 2012). *Pavano* is a "literary parodic language of the
Paduan countryside dialect," the one adopted by "pavano" poets (my thanks to
Profs Paccagnella and Piermario Vescovo for the distinction).]

I.1 The *Treatise* and Other Works on a Sober Life

"I similarly entrust to my commisioners mentioned above the treatises written by me on the conservation of the lagoons in Venice, on the reclamation of marshlands, and the one on a regulated life, thought for some time to benefit the Republic; my wanting above all that this treatise on a regulated life be printed as soon as possible for the public benefit of mortal beings." So writes Alvise Cornaro in his first will, drawn up in November 1552, "iacens in lecto infirmus corpora, sanus tamen mente ac recte loquens" [lying in my bed, weak of body, yet healthy of mind and clear as well in what I say], he resolves to convey his last wishes to his descendants.[1] It is the first direct confirmation of the existence of a treatise on sobriety, which already at the time must have circulated in a manuscript form, and which Cornaro deemed worthy for distribution, to be passed along for the benefit of mankind.

Cornaro had discovered the sober life some thirty years before, when at the age of forty, after five long years of illness, he resolved to cure himself by placing his trust exclusively in his own common sense and self-knowledge: "medicating myself," as he will say on other occasions, "on my own, in a natural way and nothing else."[2] The success of his discovery, confirmed on a daily basis by his perfect health, convinces him of the absolute *bontà* [healthiness] of an ordered life, and he soon becomes a tireless prophet; but as with all prophets, he went unheeded for quite some time, even among his most faithful friends and family members. We clearly see it in the "response" that Ruzzante indirectly gives him in his *Lettera a Marco Alvarotto* [letter to M.A.], when he presents *Madonna*

---

1 Cf. Paolo Sambin, "I testamenti di Alvise Cornaro," in *Italia Medioevale e Umanistica*, IX (1966), pp. 295–385, at p. 370 and 371. The history of A. Cornaro's testaments is not as simple as it may appear. Among the texts we have: (1) the autograph exordium undated and cancelled, in which Cornaro says he is 73 years old, can be traced back to 1551, perhaps following the incident of the carriage recounted in the *Treatise*; (2) an undated autograph draft where Cornaro claims to be seventy-four years old, taken up again with some changes, and a notable omission in the text by the notary Gaspare Villani on 22 November 1552, which attests Cornaro's first "winter" illness (winter 1552–1553); (3) the autograph will of 25 January 1555 delivered to the notary by Cornaro, "sannus per gratia Dei mente et corpore, sedens apud ignem" two days later; (4) the codicil dated 28 October 1556 in the hand of the notary; and (5) the will of 25 April 1566 written in Cornaro's still steady hand "iacens in lecto in camera solitae suae ressidentiae, sannus mente et intellectu ac rectae loquens, licet corpore senior et egritudine infirmus."

2 [*Scritti ...,*] Lettera X, from late 1554.

Allegrezza [My Lady Happiness] as the only one who "lets man live for years, who prolongs lives, adding length and breadth to life, and is not one of those women from around here with a strange sounding name." It is logical to think of Cornaro's *Ternità* [ternary] being formed of the "most rare Lady, and much loved by him, Lady Continence, mother of the Lady of Virtue, Lady of the Regulated Life, whose daughter is the beautiful Lady of Health."[3] It is no wonder then that Cornaro, convinced of having found a way to live at least one hundred years and being certain that death "before one's time" was exclusively due to the overindulgences of a disordered life, blamed the death of Ruzzante on the hated crapula.[*]

In the famous letter to Speroni, dated 2 April 1542, he mentions the death of Beolco [Ruzzante] as proof of what he was alleging, and openly expresses his bitterness at being an unheeded prophet:

> I search for some way to have my friends believe that the bodily disorders that men have, cause these men to die young. I tell them this but they do not believe me. And even if not from disorders, they die and leave me in this misery where I find myself, and even more so after the death of our dearest Messer Ruzzante, which also would have killed me from extreme sorrow, if this could kill a man, and before my having reached the age of ninety. But it was not able, because order has made me immortal and has seen to it that at the age of fifty-eight I look to be about thirty-five years old, and every day this order makes it possible for one who is ill to regain his health through simple order. I say and I predicate each of these things every day but I am not believed, and this alone saddens me, for I could be the happiest man in the world.[4]

From Speroni, Cornaro seeks the reason as to why he is not believed:

> I have no other opposition to my happiness if not for the [premature] death of my friends, who die because they do not believe me and so keep me in continuing misery. (158)[**]

---

3 [*Scritti* ...,] Lettera al Magn. Messer Aluvise (lett.V).

* [Crapula – the ill effect of drinking or eating in excess – exists as the same word in English. On crapula, see "Note on Translation," and see *Sober* ..., p. 76n9.]

4 [*Sober* ..., Letter III, p. 155;] *Scritti* ..., Lettera III.

** [Parenthetical numbers inserted in the "Introduction" refer to pages here in the Da Ponte edition.]

We do not know Speroni's response, although we do know that his ideas were entirely different from those of his interlocutor, as he will demonstrate twenty years later in the letter better known as the *Discorso contro la sobrietà* [discourse against sobriety].[5]

Approximately one year later, Cornaro, writing to his namesake the Grand Commander of Cyprus, asks of him, with the same rhetorical expedience adopted in his letter to Speroni, to find in that far-off island the formula he had searched for throughout all of Italy in vain:

> and the recipe is this: to have my friends believe that a disordered life and disorders cause infirmities and early death, since it is the conclusion held and approved of by medical schools. And since they do not believe me, they do not act [on it] and often become ill and die on me, which leaves me extremely unhappy, so that if I were to have a recipe I would conserve the few that remain to me, and be most happy, because I want for nothing else, thus thankful to the Glorious and Great Lord.[6]

Letters, like this one sent to the Magnificent Aluvise [the Commander], are the chosen means by which Cornaro communicates his discovery beyond his narrow circle of familiars, offering himself and his long and happy life as its proof. These letters are still not – as will be the ones to follow – the brief compendium of the treatise already written, so much as premises for a first draft. To the Magnificent Aluvise, Cornaro in fact speaks about his treatises on architecture and agriculture, the one completed and the other still in progress. But in regard to the one on the sober life, we find only the counterpoint between a positive Ternary (continence, regulated life, health) and negative Ternary (crapula, lust, gambling). From the latter group, only crapula appears in the definitive treatise, which leads us to believe that the first drafts were significantly different from the final one.

Mention, however vague, of the "loving memories" sent by Cornaro is found in a letter to Cardinal Sant'Angelo dated 22 April 1552:[7] it may refer to the version of the *Vita Sobria e Regolata* [a regulated and sober life] recommended in the will dated only a few months later. In January 1554, Cornaro announces having written the three treatises, but does not send any copy. On 27 January 1554, Cardinal Alvise Cornaro writes:

---

5 [See *Sober*..., p. 140] *Scritti*..., Lettera XXIV.

6 *Scritti*..., Lettera IV, to Alvise Cornaro Grand Commander of Cyprus. The letter is subsequent to May 1543 and probably goes back to the first part of the following year.

7 [*Scritti*...,] Lettera VII.

The world can yet expect from [your] *prudentia* and fine brilliance, great results, and great benefit to the everlasting honour and glory of your name and of your House, since Your Magnificence did promise me, here in this letter, three beautiful and worthy works written on Architecture, on Agriculture and on a Sober and Regulated Life; treatises that I will be awaiting with the greatest desire (…) I therefore pray Your *Magnificentia* most heartily of your wanting to hasten to put the final touches to your works, so that [your] value and virtue may be better known to the World.[8]

In May of that year, writing to his friend Domenico Morosini, Cornaro claims to have written ten treatises, but in the list written by him there are only eight, with the following subdivisions: "useful to the homeland," five, and "useful to others," three. The latter are those on *Agriculture,* "very useful and helpful," the one on *Architecture,* "very beautiful and fitting," and the one on a *Vita Regolata e Sobria,* wherein he demonstrated "what can be done, and by anyone."[9]

One might ask why Cornaro would prefer to circulate the treatises as manuscript copies and would not think instead to have them published. It is difficult to find a convincing answer: perhaps he did not wish to incur an expense not always easily recouped, or perhaps he did not like to feel deprived of the possibility of making changes to his text, expanding or condensing it, depending on the person to whom it was addressed.

Further proof of Cornaro's lack of interest in having them published is seen in the letter to the person identified only as Padre Francesco di Milano – unfortunately not dated, but presumably between 1555 and 1556 – which accompanies a copy of his treatise on the sober life, the one he gives to the priest to have printed for the purpose of keeping crapula far from Milan:

O Very Reverend Father, what joy it brings me knowing you shall be the one to return a beautiful long life to men and to their souls, a life eternal! Because that bestial and lethal crapula had deprived them of one and the other, so that by the age of 40 years they became old and died, and they would still be prosperous at 80, the way they were before the French brought this vice to Italy: where that city [Milan] became the first. And since this vice is like a contagious disease, it spread through all other cities

---

8 [*Scritti …,*] Lettera VIII.

9 [*Scritti …,*] Lettera IX. He also mentions his 10 treatises in the letter to Cardinal Sant'Angelo and Cardinal Cornaro – on 5 February 1557 (Lettera XIV) – without, however, specifying any subject.

and locales in Italy and now, freed as [Milan] will be of it, which was the
first, all others will follow what they do.[10]

Mention of the French as the importers of crapula – not found in the
published text or in his subsequent writings – would appear to be from
certain parts of a draft different from the definitive one.

Who, or what, induced Cornaro, so reluctant to publish his writings, to
entrust the treatise to the presses of Grazioso Percacino, at the time the
best printer in Padua? For the edition of works by Ruzzante, Cornaro had
first turned to Gabriel Giolito (the *Piovana* is from 1548) who had dedicated the brief work to him [Cornaro],[11] with each of the subsequent
ones to Stefano Alessi, and began printing them in 1551. Perhaps it was
being able to avail himself of a printer within the same city that made
him choose Percacino, who had opened his shop only several years before (1554), but above all for how well he had acquitted himself, in 1556,
in printing the two orations to the Venetian Inquisitors and the *Consiglio
sopra la peste di Venetia* [advice on the Venetian plague] by the illustrious
physician and philosopher Bernardino Tomitano, a very close friend of
Cornaro.[12] In any case, the prior decision – that of having the treatise
printed – must not have been either a simple or an easy one. Nothing is
known with any certainty, but several indications and coincidences have
opened up a few possibilities. First of all, there is the fact that the *Treatise*

---

10 [*Scritti …,*] Lettera XII.
11 But this is more likely an independent initiative by Giolito, who, on 29 August 1547
   had asked the Senate for the right to print the *Vaccaria* and the *Piovana*, see Emilio
   Lovarini, *Studi sul Ruzzante e la letteratura pavana*, ed. G. Folena (Padua 1965),
   pp. 162–3. The dedication by Giolito is in [*Scritti …,*] *Appendice* III 3.
12 A reference to the orations cited in note 4 of the *Trattato* and of the *Consiglio de l'Eccell.
   M. Bernardino Tomitano sopra la peste di Vinetia l'anno MDLVI. Al Magnifico M. Francesco
   Longo del Clarissimo M. Antonio* (Padua: Appresso Gratioso Percacino 1556). It is no
   coincidence that in 1558, perhaps some months before the *Treatise*, Percacino printed
   the first book of *Rime* by the *pavano* poets Magagnò, Menon, and Begotto. As Magagnò
   recalls: "A' dissi: 'Qui versitti, / Che solea zà cantar barba Begotto, / E Menon, c'ha
   sì dolce el sigolotto, / Se perderà debotto, / Se vu, Segnor, no fè ch'a' possa anare /
   Dal Prechacin a fargi intorcolare.'" [Thus he said: Those poor verses, / that once were
   sung by uncle Begotto / and Menon, who played the flute so well, / will soon be lost /
   if you, Signori, do not see to it that I may go / to Percacino to have them sent to press]
   (vv. 78–81, [fol.] 24v).
   In addition to his writings on the sober life, Cornaro publishes only two other brief
   works, both in 1560 and still with Percacino: the *Aricordo del modo che si ha da tenere, per
   fare che il fiume Musone con la Brenta vadi al mare per il porto di Chioza*, and the *Trattato di
   acque*.

appears with the dedication by Tomitano to Bishop Cornelio Musso, the beloved friend and "virtual son" to Cornaro, from which we learn that, knowing full well "the honest desire by the Author" (72), Tomitano took on the task "to make known under your honoured name this brief work no less beautiful than it is enjoyable, no less enjoyable than it is beneficial to the world."[13]

It is owing to the affectionate insistence by Tomitano, therefore, and to his ability to call upon their common friendship with Musso that Cornaro conceded; but other arguments, perhaps less incisive, though just as convincing overall, must have been brought to bear. Tomitano, in his capacity as a physician, was perfectly aware of what was occurring within the academic world at the time, where discussions had long been raging in regard to a method to achieve perfect health and to prolong life, also as a consequence of the ongoing occurrences of pestilence that were devastating cities.[14] At the time, new treatises were always being printed, going back to classical ones in the original or, more often, in translation; in 1548, in Venice, for example, the *De Vita* [*Three Books on Life*] by Marsilio Ficino came out [in Latin] along with its translation [in Italian].[15] In 1554, again in Venice, dietary rules were reintroduced that had been written a century before by Michele Savonarola* for Borso d'Este;[16] not to mention the works by Galen and their translations, one

---

13 [*Sober ...*, p. 72]; *Scritti ...*, pp. 75–6.

14 For more on pestilence, see "Venezia e la peste 1348/1797," Venice, 1979, in the interesting "Catalogue" [*Alvise Cornaro e il suo tempo*, Padua 1980] from the Cornaro exhibit.

15 *Marsilio Ficino fiorentino filosofo eccellentissimo de le tre Vite, cioè, A qual guisa si possono le persone letterate mantenere in sanità. Per qual guisa si possa l'huomo prolungare la vita. Con che arte, e mezzi ci possiamo quest asana, e la lunga vita prolungare per uia del cielo. Recato tutto di latino in buona lingua uolgare.* At the end: (In Venetia per Michel Tramezzino, MDXLVIII) [cited herein as *Tre Vite ...,*].

 * [Giovanni Michele Savonarola (1385?–1464?) was a physician at the Este court, humanist, professor at the University of Padua, a renowned scholar on gynecology, pediatrics, and diet; he also wrote in the vernacular, *Libreto de tute le cosse che se manzano: un libro dietetica,* [book on all the things to eat: a dietetic book.] His grandson was Girolamo Savonarola (1452–1498), the Dominican monk who, in 1498, was hung and simultaneously burned at the stake in the Piazza della Signoria in Florence on the charge of heresy as decreed by Pope Alexander VI.]

16 *Trattato utilissimo di molte regole, per conseruare la sanità, dichiarando qual cose siano utili da mangiare, & quali triste; & medesimamente di quelle che si beuono per Italia. Aggiontoui alcuni dubii molto notabili,* Venetii, per gli heredi di Giouanne Paduano (1554). See the critical edition, edited by Jane Nystedt, *Libreto de tute le cosse che se manzano. Un libro di dietica di Michele Savonarola, medico padovano del secolo XV* (Stockholm 1982).

of which is *Delli mezzi che si possono tenere per conservarci la sanità* [on ways to conserve our health] that appeared in Venice in 1549.[17] Cornaro, on the other hand, did not want his *Treatise* to be known as a medical study and Tomitano clearly states this, almost as if to prevent possible accusations on the part of the distrustful and prickly professors at the University of Padua:

> Nevertheless, let every man know who will read of these things that I do not publish this volume as a physician nor as a medical book, given that the Author has never practised this art as a profession. Nor was it his intention to enrich the vast Ocean of Medicine with this small current of his branch, as it was something he knew very well had not been overlooked by more than one classical writer, that is, in elaborating and in broadening the terms of this art. (73)

Cornaro's polemic against physicians comes through in all the works: he does not have "authors," and he never cites examples or sources, the only probative example being himself and his own longevity. The usefulness of physicians is not put in question, but they serve only for those who do not follow a sober life; and in any case, they lack the power to prolong the lives of the *sensuali*.*

Along with classical medical works, a new treatise had come out in Venice in 1550, the work of the famous physician and philologist, Tommaso Rangone, under the captivating title *De vita homini ultra CXX annos protrahenda* [how men may live beyond 120 years]:[18] an imposing work in which, by means of an unbelievable number of citations – from disparate texts and authors ranging from the Bible to the Fathers of the Church, ancient physicians to Latin and Greek classical works, with a few rare examples, somewhat unconvincing, of personal experiences – Rangone demonstrates that the natural end to human life is at one hundred and twenty years. The work was an immediate success, because the author published a part of it in [an Italian] translation under the title *Consiglio*

---

17 Galen, *Delli mezzi che si possono tenere per conseruarci la sanità. Recato in questa lingua nostra da M. Giouanni Tarcagnota.* At the end: (In Venetia per Michele Tramezzino, MDXLIX) [cited herein as *Delli mezzi …,*].

 * [*sensuali*: "sensual," as a substantive also in English signifies one (like an animal) seeking only to satisfy sense driven needs. See *Sober …*, p. 81n19.]

18 *Iulio III Sanctissimo. Thomae Philologi Ravenna De uita homini ultra CXX. annos protahenda. Cardinalis De Monte auspiciis* (Venetiis Sanctissimi Iubilei 1550).

come i Venetiani possano vivere sempre sani [advice on how Venetians can live always in good health],[19] but it was later forgotten. We remember it now only because it served as an incentive for Cornaro and reinforced his conviction that the limit to human life conceded by God was very long for everyone, and man should end his days gently "out of resolution" of the humours in his body.

Cornaro is careful not to cite Rangone directly, but it is no coincidence that in the letter to Speroni he would say that he could not die, since he had not yet reached ninety years, and that, in the one to the Grand Commodore (1554), he was sure he would not fall ill and die for another thirty years (he admitted to being sixty at the time). Whereas in the *Compendio* [*Compendium*] (1561), he claims that men "would have lived to one hundred, the end conceded by God and by our own Mother Nature to us her sons,"[20] and in the *Amorevole Essortatione* [*Loving Exhortation*] (1565) he maintains that if they had "begun a life of order and sobriety, they would have grown older, as I have done, being well conditioned. And they, having been born by the Grace of the Great Lord with such a good and perfect complexion, would live to one hundred and twenty years, just as others have done who maintained a sober life, which we hear about everywhere."[21] In December 1559, he had written to [Zan Paolo] da Ponte:

> And I am confident and certain I can no longer die if not from a natural death, which is from resolution, once having passed the age of the one hundred years conceded and terminated by God and by our own Mother Nature to man, who does not overlook conserving his life as I have done.[22]

His reading of Rangone, if nothing else, had led him to push back the ultimate finish line by some thirty years.

Now convinced by his friend to publish his treatise, Cornaro set out to prepare the definitive text. We are in the final months of 1557 or the

---

19 (In Venetia per Francesco de Patriarchi 1565). The date suggests an attempt on the part of Rangone to recuperate the success that Cornaro had taken away from him. Rangone, who died in Venice on 13 September 1577, at "only" ninety-four years of age, had the sculptor Alessandro Vittoria make a statue of him for the entranceway to the Church of San Giuliano with the bilingual inscription, in Greek and Hebrew, that memorialized him as being the discoverer of the method for living long.

20 [*Sober ...*, p. 107] *Scritti ...*, p. 106.

21 [*Sober ...*, pp. 125–6] *Scritti ...*, p. 123.

22 [*Sober ...*, p. 172] *Scritti ...*, Lettera XVII.

early part of 1558: the time is construed from what he says about his grandsons Giacomo Alvise and Piero, to whom he attributes the ages of eighteen and two years, respectively, while in 1558 they were nineteen and three: Giacomo Alvise was born 13 September 1539, and Piero on 20 March 1555.[23] With the draft finalized, Cornaro passes the manuscript to Tomitano, who, undoubtedly with the full consent of the author, very discreetly intervenes in regard to the text – correcting various dissonant wordings and somewhat dated writing style and revising the punctuation – or so it would seem on first impression in comparing [it to] other publications and the autograph letters. However, even the editor misses the strange mistake, rather the amazing incongruence within the text, which only eighteenth-century publishers, alerted by Cicogna, will quietly do away with: the matter of the differing ages that Cornaro attributes to himself, first by saying he is eighty-one years old (78) – reconfirmed when he speaks about the illness he had four years before at the age of seventy-eight (86) – then maintaining to be eighty-three years of age, exactly ten years more than the Greek, who, at the age of seventy-three, wrote a tragedy (97).

The *Trattato de la Vita Sobria,* a booklet 18.5 × 14 cm in size, printed on quality paper in beautiful italic characters, was published by the Percacino presses in November 1558, and was such an immediate success that within a few months it was worthy of a pirated edition, prepared by a Venetian publisher as anonymous as he was sly. At that time, copyright laws were unknown and the author or printer could only petition the Senate of the Serenissima* for the privilege of printing a work over a certain number of years. However, not even the assiduous Venetian laws were enough to defeat the cases of fraud in the publishing field; instead, works by even well-known authors were often printed under the name of another held to be more marketable. Such is the case for example of the *Rhodiana* by Andrea Calmo, which becomes the work of Ruzzante in the edition done by Domenico de Farri in 1561 and in those to follow.

---

23 Cf. the genealogical tree provided by F.L. Maschietto, *Elena Lucrezia Conaro Piscopia (1646–1684) prima donna laureata nel mondo* [*the first woman in the world to obtain a university degree*] (Padua 1978), in which appears a mysterious twelfth grandson by the name of Pietro Bernardo Giuseppe, born 20 March 1553, that is, exactly seven months after the birth of Girolamo. If this is not the same Piero cited by us, as one would suspect from the strange coincidence of date and name, thought must then be given to an aborted birth or an infant who died shortly after birth.

 * [La Serenissima = Venice Her Most Serene Republic.]

The Venetian printing of the *Treatise*, in a smaller format and using a paper and typeface of a more current font, is a copy, with some graphic variations and corrections made to several obvious errors in printing overlooked in the *princeps*, and states that it was printed "*A San Luca al Segno del Diamante*," [via San Luca under the Mark of the Diamond] without the date or name of the publisher.

It would be interesting to know how many copies of the two editions were printed, although we believe it must have been relatively high for the times, in as much as the two texts are not considered "rare" publications.

In regard to the content of the work, we will let the author speak and explain it in a few lines:

> Seeing them filled with such honest desire, and in order to help them, together with others who wish to read my discourse, I will write on it, stating the reasons that forced me to abandon crapula and to embrace a sober life, recounting the entire method I followed in doing so, and relating how that good habit then operated in me. It will thus be clearly understood how easy it is to be rid of the abuse of crapula; and in conclusion, I will include the many uses and benefits to be had from a sober life. (78–9)

Cornaro's argument is very simple: sobriety is the only perfect solution to the physical and psychic ills of man, because from it are derived serenity and happiness, and the fear of death and that of final judgment are removed. The order Cornaro proposes is natural, it belongs to the laws of nature and reflects divine order; therefore, crapula, which is disorder, not only destroys human life but puts society itself in danger. As we know, these ideas are not new; what is new is the confident and conversational way they are expressed. And what is inspired is the way in which the author offers himself up as an indisputable example of what he believes, in addition to the comforting assurance of someone who bases his own experience on facts and not on words.

It does not matter if, to give credence to his thesis, Cornaro is forced to resort to the risky expedient of exaggerating his age, which can be taken as a laughable failing of old age, but which, instead, is a completely calculated choice, and perhaps in the end a difficult one. What matters is that this not very "clever" frabrication enabled him to build credibility among his readers up to the present day. No one can remember Tommaso Rangone – who only and always relied on the words of others – and yet he died at the age of ninety-four years. But we continue to speak of Cornaro, even though we now know that he did not even reach his original goal of ninety years.

After the release of the *Treatise*, Cornaro sent, as was customary, various copies to friends and admirers, and in return he received their appreciation and praise; something that to us seems rather overblown but it was part of the social rules of the time. Belonging to this period is the letter by Paolo Pino,[24] who, for the occasion, took the trouble of taking texts sacred and profane and putting together Dante and Epicurus on the exaltation of sobriety; but as to overstating, Cornaro does no less for himself when he writes [Zan Paulo] da Ponte in December 1559 about the great success of his *Treatise* on German soil:

> Moreover, day by day there are new joys for me, since my treatise on the sober life, known throughout different places, has operated for the reasons now discussed, in as much as Germany has begun to ban excessive drinking. It is what men were doing by inviting each other [to drink] and viewing it as a virtuous [manly] act, when it is a dissolute and fatal one. Many of my friends and acquaintances from these neighbouring areas thank me, some by letter and some in person, for the useful guidance given them in that treatise.[25]

The exaggeration is much too obvious for us to dwell on. But what would Cornaro have said, had he known that at a distance of two centuries his treatise would have saved the life of an English miller, and that the case would have been written up in medical journals of the time?[26]

That the brief work will have an immediate appeal to the reader is a certainty, and that over the years it will solicit commentaries and spark debates among noted physicians or the average reader is amply demonstrated. It was in response to objections raised from many sides that Cornaro would decide to publish over time other writings on the sober life. We do not have any documentation in this regard [of the objections], with the exception of the letter by Speroni in 1562; but Cornaro himself – in these things always very attentive and precise – states the arguments of his adversaries before offering his own reply.

---

24 Lettera XVI [*Sober …*, p. 167].

25 Lettera XVII [*Sober …*, p. 173].

26 M. Milani, "Come raggiungere l'immortalità vivendo cent'anni, ovvero La fortuna della *Vita Sobria* nel mondo anglosassone," in *Cultura Neolatina* 40 (1980), pp. 333–56. [See "How to Attain Immortality Living One Hundred Years, or, The Fortune of the *Vita Sobria* in the Anglo-Saxon World", (cited herein as "Immortality …,") *Sober …*, p. 183].

Within a few months of the release of the *Treatise*, Cornaro feels the need to intervene with a brief text, printed on both the recto and verso of a single sheet 28 × 18 cm in size, under the title *Aggionta al Trattato de la Vita Sobria di me Luigi Cornaro* [*Addition to the Treatise on the Sober Life by me, Luigi* Cornaro*]; there is no date, location or printer, but judging from the font and style of pagination, we can confidently attribute it to Percacino. For us, the material presents an absolutely new development, because it was never reprinted and was not noticed by any scholar prior to us; this is surprising, since the *Addition* can be found included with the *Treatise* and *Loving Exhortation* in a miscellany at the Biblioteca del Seminario of Padua.[27]

The *Addition* opens with the realization – written in a tone of one who marvels at the fact – that after the *Treatise* had been issued, no one had yet taken up the sober life:

And though it is praised by all, it was nonetheless avoided by all, almost ab-
horred, as if it were depraved and not the daughter of blessed and virtuous
Continence, born of Divine Reason; a special grace conceded to man by
Our Lord so that he might be different and superior to brute animals. (102)

He thus decides to look for more receptive ears, turning to the "elderly, who ordinarily suffer all of the time – some with the pain of gout, of their side, or catarrh, and of other similar illnesses deemed as incurable – hoping that at least these, to free themselves of those, would make themselves my companions and attempt to become healthy" (102), in the same way as he had done.

The contradiction in what was said to da Ponte is evident, but at the same time, here we see reflected two fundamental objections: one by those who claim they were unable to live with the restricted diet proposed by him because they would not have been able to enjoy so little food, "therefore, not enjoying it, they would fall into mortal weakness": and one by those who denied that sobriety has the ability to prolong

---

* [Luigi = Alvise. See "Terminology": *Alvise*.]

27 A manuscript copy of 1845, done by the Paduan, A. Mussato, is part of the edition of
the *Discorsi* edited by Bartolomeo Gamba in 1826 at the Biblioteca Civica at Padua.
The accompanying letter that Mussato included with the edition is provided in the
[*Scritti* …,] appendix. On the history of Cornaro's writings, see Milani, "Appunti su
Alvise Cornaro e la *Vita Sobria* in margine a una mostra a lui dedicate," in *Giornale
Storico della letteratura Italiana* 159 (1982), pp. 216–44.

life, "which (as they say) is determined for man at his birth and has a preset end." To the first point, Cornaro responds that taste, ruined by too much food, will return "to its proper nature" within a few days after starting the diet; to the second, he repeats that "they should not judge that end to be absolutely determined, but – being that it is their death – as the resolution of the regulated [body] prescribed by the Divine Mind; [a prescription] which does not necessarily operate, however, and just as predestination is conditioned – as the Holy Scriptures teach – so too this end is conditional" (104). Nothing seems to scratch the surface of Conaro's confidence:

> I thus conclude that mine will not be death (…) but the separation of these two junctures, from which will come pure resolution; whence can be seen by the aforementioned benefits and indications that I am a long way from death. Resolution will therefore come to those who maintain a sober life, which is easy to do for the reasons I have demonstrated and for the experience that can be seen in me, a mere man. And I affirm that a sober life is a cheerful and enjoyable one to implement; hence, I would neither write nor reason so heartily on it if not for my great desire to be helpful. (105)

Not even the death of his son-in-law has the power to shake his faith: the sober life, as he had already said in regard to the death of Ruzzante, consents to bearing even the greatest sufferings with serenity:

> Neither the death of my son-in-law, which leaves me with the great responsibility of becoming a father in his place to his eleven children, could diminish part of my generosity or a single particle of reason that is in me, nor the loss of an acquisition that I could have made of 150 thousand ducats, lost to me because my women had little understanding of it; or for having lost the lawsuit selected to be overseen by them contrary to my way of thinking. So it is that all three of these extraordinary and very damaging incidents had no power to diminish my spirit or my happiness or my contentment.[28]

It is surprising to find grouped here such diverse misfortunes, but similar levelling experiences serve Cornaro to demonstrate in depth, at whatever the cost, the justification of his own claims, because the image he has patiently and wilfully constructed of his persona cannot

---

28 [*Sober* …, p. 171–2; *Scritti* …,] Lettera XVII to [Zan Paulo] da Ponte.

tolerate the least hint of suspicion. The death at only forty-five years of age of his son-in-law, a man of utmost intelligence, most gentle demeanour, and of singular integrity – citing the words of Piero Valeriano[29] – was even less imputable to crapula and to disorders than that of Ruzzante, and it also provided negative proof against Cornaro's theories; but he appears not to take any notice and does not confront the issue. However, we will find mention of it in the third text to follow shortly thereafter.

The *Compendio breve de la Vita Sobria* [*Brief Compendium of the Sober Life*], issued in 1561 by the usual Percacino [press], presents itself as a well-honed summary of the treatise, to which were added a series of responses to the questions it had provoked. By then, the *Vita sobria* had begun to benefit a number of people, especially those "born with a poor complexion," and Cornaro now aims to convince those "born with a good [one]," who, even after fifty years of age continue along with a disordered life, thereby procuring their death before reaching man's golden age into his eighties: "I had wanted" – he rationalizes at the end of the piece – "to keep this addition to my Treatise to a few words, but for other reasons: because a lengthy read is seen by a few, while a short one is seen by many and I would like many to read it and so benefit those many" (116).

The arguments Cornaro rebuts in the *Compendium* are not of a philosophical nature: he limits his responses, in a calm and convincing manner, to the objections that deal exclusively with the diet proposed by him. As to the problem of whether or not sobriety does or does not prolong life, he resolves it by simply placing his trust in common sense:

> We respond that we know who prolonged his life in the past, and we know that I prolong it now. It cannot then be said that a sober life shortens it, since infirmity shortens it; and so there is no doubt that this does not shorten life. It is thus better to live being healthy at all times than to live being ill many times, in order to conserve one's radical humour; by which we can reasonably conclude that the sacred Sober Life may be the true mother of health and long life. (113)

---

29 Valeriano dedicates the XLI book of his *Hieroglyphica* to Giovanni Cornaro Piscopia; see [in *Scritti* ...,] *Appendice*, VII I. Bishop Musso will say in a letter to Chiara: "And in which canton in Italy is the valour of [your] Consort not known, and the integrity and love by which Your Ladyship has lived with him?" [*Scritti* ...,] p. 242.

The shadow of his son-in-law's death does not disturb the serene equilibrium of the old prophet: for this also figures, as did the death of his brother Giacomo and that of Ruzzante, within the laws of a disordered life:

> O unhappy and miserable life, my enemy, you know only to kill those who follow you! The many very dear relatives and friends you have killed are the ones, who, not believing me because of you, I could now be enjoying! But you could not kill me although you would have willingly done so, and in spite of you I am alive. And so I have come to that advanced age. (115)

Copies of the *Compendium* occasionally included with the *Treatise*, were sent with a letter of accompaniment to friends and important personages. Cornaro was planning to send them to princes and dukes, as well, however the accompanying letter was left as a rough draft.[30] Among the friends who receive the writings is Mario Savorgnan, who immediately responds with a long and fascinating letter in which he speaks about a little of everything and says he is willing to follow the teachings of Cornaro.[31] Of a very different tone, however, is the reply from Sperone Speroni, who uses his copy of the *Compendium* as an occasion for a point-by-point rebuttal of Cornaro's thesis, arriving at the definition of the much exalted "death by resolution" to be a senseless death by starvation.[32] Bartolomeo Zacco, instead, declares himself convinced by Cornaro's reasoning, but he asks him to explain why, despite the writings of many sages, the world always continues along the same path.[33]

Also falling among the "accompanying works" is the letter to Daniele Barbaro, the Patriarch Elect of Aquileia, who at the time was attending meetings at the Council of Trent. Cornaro then had the letter printed, which came out in September 1563. It is in praise of reason and of experience versus the hopelessly long-winded academics in Padua:

> and so you see, Lordship, how men can fool themselves with their own opinions when they are not founded on a real foundation. (120)

---

30 [*Scritti* ...,] Lettera XXI. In all probability the undated draft is from 1562.

31 [*Scritti* ...,] Lettera XXII.

32 [*Sober* ..., p. 144] *Scritti* ..., Lettera XXIV. Speroni writes to a friend in September 1563: "I thank you for the sympathy for my pain, in which I too will [carry on] as others do. I am almost too healthy, since I live too long, because one who lives too long, is one who sees his dearest die, and in this I believe to be right, contrary to the Magnificent Alvise Cornaro, that if God conserves in me the things remaining, I will glady live a few days more ...." (copy in the T. XI of the Speroni MSS at the Biblioteca Vescovile of Padua).

33 [*Scritti* ...,] Lettera XXVII.

For the "many excellent Physicians of those who teach at this University – philosophers as much as doctors," Cornaro speaks of giving an actual lesson and in the end of having fully convinced them. In the latter part of the text, he defends the *Treatise* from the accusation of being a useless work for being impracticable, and he finishes with a categorical assertion destined to be disproved in a most drammatic manner only a few months later:

> And if it was the [end] that they say, which is one whereby a man dies before his time, it would then be by a Partial and Unjust God depriving a person of life before his time, and not allowing him to enjoy the most perfect age, which is once he has passed eighty years. Because this is an age full of reason, experience, knowledge, goodness and charity, free of sin and therefore much beloved by God. We must believe that He would want every man to enjoy that age, and it is to this outcome that He gave to man reason and intellect that with these he could arrive at that age – but man does not want to give up his sensuality nor taste nor appetites, and will therefore die before his time. (123)

Never has Cornaro been so explicit and extreme: if in the *Treatise* he had portrayed himself as God the Father surrounded by a heavenly host, now he assumes the aura of the Inflexible Justice of the Eternal [Father]. The Heavens do not make him wait long for a response: within the first months of the following year, Fantino, his second-born grandson, dies; in July, Ferigo dies, the third of those grandchildren "all the most beautiful, all the most healthy," of whom Cornaro had taken so much pride. Fantino was twenty-three years old, Ferigo twenty-two.

The terrible blow is reflected in his last writing, the *Amorevole Essortatione* [*Loving Exhortation*], issued around May 1565, exactly one year before his death, and here, the grand old man speaks on death with extreme and enviable serenity. He still praises the sober life, his happiness in being able to write and help his "dear Homeland," and to witness the success of his treatises. Free of every passion and perturbation of his soul, he remains undisturbed by the thought of death:

> nor can the death of my grandsons or other relatives or friends upset me if not as a first impulse, but it is soon gone; and the losses of my business dealings upset me even less (as many have seen to their great admiration). (127)

Yet, for the first time in his long life, he is forced to modify his theory, implicitly recognizing that more powerful than a sober life are the "revolutions of the Heavens," that is to say: destiny. It is not, therefore, the Will of God – which here is left unnamed – nor that of Nature, but an unknown reason that governs human life and there is nothing to do but take note:

> I would say, therefore, that some are born so scarcely alive they live only a few days or months or years, and it is not well understood if the cause of so short a life comes from a defect of the father or of the mother in conceiving him, or the revolutions of the Heavens, or a defect of Nature, which still comes from those Heavens; and so I can never believe that, being the Mother of everyone, she could be partial about her children. Therefore, not being able to know the cause is to rely by necessity on what everyday can be seen as fact. Others are born quite lively and healthy, but with a poor and weak complexion, and some among these live to the age of ten, some to twenty, others to thirty or forty years, but none reach an old age. (125)

The *Loving Exhortation*, which also deals at some length on the not entirely sober life of the religious, Cornaro sends, as was his custom, to competent readers, among whom are the Bishops Bollani of Brescia and Cornaro of Bergamo, in addition to Gabriele Cornaro and the knight, Giovanni da Leze, another living example of grand longevity.[34]

I.2 The Regulations of Cornaro and Search for a "Long Life"

Man, according to medical theory at the time, is composed of four elements: air, fire, water, and earth; these elements correspond to the four humours, having the [respective] properties of blood, bile, phlegm, and black bile. The predominance of one humour over another gives rise to the "temperaments" [complexions] – sanguine, choleric, phlegmatic, and melancholic – each having their own characteristics that are reflected in the physical aspect of the person. Every man, knowing his temperament, will be able to regulate his own life according to the exact dietary norms that medical science – beginning with Hippocrates

---

34 [*Scritti* ...,] Lettere XXX, XXXI, XXXVI.

and Galen – has indentified and prescribed.[35] When the humours are perfect, in agreement, and proportional, and left undisturbed by external causes – man is healthy. Only a "perturbation of the humours" can provoke an illness, and the cure will, in that case, consist in having them return to their original calm [equilibrium].[36] The only substantial difference among men is due to having been born with either a good or poor complexion, that is, a strong or weak one: the former will have a healthy and long life, the latter, a short life troubled by much illness.

It is on this fundamental point where the originality of Cornaro is fully realized. As is evident, he does not accept this banal truism but is absolutely convinced that even the weakest and most sickly complexion could, by living soberly, reach an extreme old age. To reduce the innovation of Cornaro to only dietetic norms – which in themselves are already

---

35 It is worth reading what the otherwise unidentified Lucio Fauno first says in the preface to his translation [from Latin into Italian] of the [*Three Books* ...,] by Marsilio Ficino: "There are, therefore (as physicians say), four humours in man, blood; *flemma*, which the Latins called pituita; bile, which the Greeks called choler; and black bile, which the same [Greeks] call melancholy. The nature of blood is air, warm and wet, and contains mixed within it the other three humours. The nature of bile is fire, warm and dry. Phlegm is water, cold and wet. Black bile is earth, cold and dry. And whoever looks closely, will see all four of these humours each time someone has blood drawn from a vein, so that the froth, or lightest part of the blood, and which goes to the top, is the choler or bile, as we call it. Phlegm is that wateriness, which flows in the manner of little streams in the blood, black bile those thick dregs that remain at the bottom of the vessel. All the rest then is blood. According to how plentifully one abounds in these humours, different effects are then seen in man, because where he is more plentiful in choler, there we see irascibility, agility, and quickness of mind; where there is more of black bile, we see timidity, little spirit, and indolence. Pituita [makes him] slow and cold. Blood [makes him] happy, cheerful and disposed to laugh. The Choleric, in respect to their heat, have straight and lean limbs, their hair is frizzy, they are dark-skinned, and their veins swollen; and to them, for the most part, it seems that while sleeping they see weapons, battles, and fiery things. The Melancholic are pale, mournful, and pensive, their veins are so narrow they are barely visible; and to them it seems they always see horrendous and frightening things in their dreams. The Phlegmatic are less hairy, have soft flesh, straight hair, and for the most part are fat; and when asleep it seems to them that they are thrown into rivers, or are swimming, and other similar things having to do with water. The Sanguine have all of the above in a moderate way, and are ruddy; and when asleep, everything appears to them in the colour red."] ([in Fauno] IV, not numbered.)

36 "That state and composition of the body, in which we do not feel any torment from our pains, nor is our life hampered in our activities – we call health" (Galen, *Delli mezzi* ..., p. 7v).

extraordinary for the times – means to trivialize Cornaro's thought overall, and in the end it does not explain either the stir that arose from his theories or the success of his work. Cornaro is not the first to establish the end for a human life at a century or beyond, as has already been pointed out, but he is the first to hold that it may be achieved by any man, no matter what his complexion might be;[37] hence, the accusations brought against him for not having taken into account the laws of nature and even of violating divine laws. And we understand better his stubborn certainty in attributing the death of many friends and relatives to crapula and to disorders, until the demise of his two grandsons will compel him to acknowledge that, even while following a sober life, one can die at twenty years of age.

Today's readers, accustomed to having their own cholesterol measured, will smile over the diet Cornaro followed:

> And these are my foods: first, bread, *panatella* or broth with an egg or other similar good soups; for meat, I eat veal, kid, and beef; I eat any sort of poultry, I eat partridge, and fowl such as thrush; I also eat fish, saltwater ones like sea-bream or similar, and from freshwater, pike and the like. These are all foods suitable for the old, and they must be content with these, not wanting more, since they are ample. (114)

He had said in the *Treatise*:

> among the bread, egg yolk, meat and soup – I ate what in all weighed twelve short [*alla sottile*] ounces (...) and (...) I drank fourteen ounces of wine. (86)

The weight in short ounces shows how meticulously he measured his food.[38] For us, such amounts are equal to 284 grams of food, and 333

---

37 Much more open to compromise, Marsilio Ficino (*De le tre vite* ..., pp. 28v–29r) had said: "This is why we are certainly right to conclude with Hippocrates that art [and the discipline] is long and we can only attain it by a long life. But a long life is not just something the Fates promise once and for all from the beginning, but something that is procured by our effort . . . . Through this foresight not only do people who are strong by nature very often attain a long life but also sometimes the weakest" [*Marsilio Ficino: Three Books on Life*. Critical Edition and Translation with Introduction and Notes by Carol V. Kaske and John R. Clark (Binghamton, NY: Medieval and Renaissance Texts & Studies in conjunction with The Renaissance Society of America, 1989), p. 511 (cited herein as *Three Books* ...,)].

38 Venetian measurements distinguished between the *lira grossa* [full pound] equal to 12 ounces of 192 carats, and the *lira sottile* [short pound] equal to 12 ounces of 122 carats. [Also see *Sober* ..., p. 86n30]

grams of wine. It is difficult to calculate the caloric value with such scarce data; in any case, keeping in mind that 100 grams of bread are equivalent to 274 calories, an egg yolk to 30 calories, 350 grams of wine to 337 calories, and that all the meat is low in calories, and calculating again for condiments, which Cornaro does not account for, we arrive at about 1,000 calories. The resulting diet is ideal for anyone of eighty years living a sedentary and tranquil life,[39] as long as Cornaro is referring to a single meal and does not mean instead the entire daily intake of food. Doubt had grown among others, including the famous [Girolamo] Cardano, who – surprised that the quantity of wine indicated by Cornaro would be superior to that of food, something contrary to all the rules – noted that

---

39 The same result is calculated by George Cooke, who says this in regard to Cornaro's diet: "Now in many respects this system is absolutely opposed to the conclusions of our modern doctors and dieticians. But, while their theories are the result of laboratory work and experiments on animals, Cornaro's diet was based on a completely successful experiment on himself (...) Of course he is only one case, and what suited him may not suit everybody, as he says himself. But I suggest that his principles deserve a close and imprejudiced examination. We may yet discover that he knew more about diet than our modern scientific authorities (...) Cornaro's diet, on the other hand, consisted of about 1,000 calories. Of course, as Cornaro himself points out, an old man needs less than a young one (...) But even so the difference is striking (...) It is clear that it is possible to keep in good health without losing weight on a diet consisting of 1,000 calories (...) And if only a few foods are used, as in Cornaro's case, it is possible that the body may be able to extract much more nourishment from them than if a large number of different articles, all mixed up together, are consumed, as usually happens at present. As regards drink Cornaro's practice is still more remarkable (...) The water in his 12 oz. of food may have amounted to about 8 oz., and his total consumption of liquids would thus be about 22 oz. a day, or just over a pint. I do not know of any other case in which a man has lived on such a small amount of liquid for so long (...) Cornaro does not say definitely that he had nothing at all to drink apart from the 14 oz. of wine but he certainly implies as much (...) The necessity of including an ample supply of fresh fuits and vegetables in one's diet, is insisted upon, nowadays, by pratically all food experts. And yet Cornaro, if we may believe his account, used no fresh fruits or vegetables at all – apart from the wine, of course (...) But Cornaro lived before the machine age, and so would necessarily use foods that were, to a large extent, in their natural condition. His bread, for example, would be stone-ground, and by this process many of the vitamins, and essential mineral salts, that are extracted in the modern methods of milling, would not be lost. In his case, fruits and vegetables would supply no essential element which he was not already getting from his other foods, and, consequently, he was, perhaps, better without them" (*How to live for a Hundred Years and Avoid Disease. A Treatise by Luigi Cornaro the Sixteenth Century Italian Centenarian.* Translated by George Herbert with an Introduction by George Cooke comparing Cornaro's System with Modern Theories of Diet (Oxford, 1935), pp. 7–31 passim).

the foods cited had different nutritive values, and concludes a little spite-
fully in the end that Cornaro seemingly spoke more as a philosopher
than as a physician.[40]

Indeed, the passage by Cornaro can leave some doubt, because his
"in all" is sufficiently vague. To resolve the question, other passages are
helpful in gleaning the fact that those few ounces comprised all of the
food. "I eat little," – he writes in the *Treatise* – "because that amount is
enough for my small and weakened stomach" (91); and he explains in
the *Addition*:

> the old need little food to conserve their life and health, since Nature is
> content with little; and that a large amount of food, because it cannot be
> digested by them, converts into repletion, which [repletion] generates ill
> humours and ill humours generate infirmities. (103)

For the elderly, it is not enough simply to eat a little; he should divide
that little amount several times, just as Nature herself demonstrates:

> since in his youth he ate twice a day, in his old age he should divide that
> daily food of two meals into four, because that food, so divided, will be more
> easily digested by his stomach (...) and continue to decrease the quantity as
> his years continue to increase. (114)

In fact, Cornaro reduced his own food little by little as he grew older
(although perhaps in this case, he did not increase his own age); in this
way, it assists Nature wanting death to be from the pure resolution of the
humours:

> seeing that my years are increasing, I therefore decrease the quantity of
> food I eat, since such a decrease is necessary; nor can one do otherwise,

---

40 Furthermore, Cardano [1501–1576] accepted without any apparent difficulty the
   idea of a daily diet: "sibi rationem vitae pondere praescripsit cibi duodecim unciarum in
   dies, potus quatuordecim" (Hieronymi Cardani Mediolanensis, Ciuisq. Bononiensis,
   Medici Clarissimi *Opus nouum cunctis de Sanitate Tuenda, ac uita producenda studiosi
   apprime necessarium: in quatuor libros digestum*. A Rodulpho Sylvestro Bononiensi
   Medico, recens in lucent editurn. Romae Anno MDLLXXX, liber iv,' 283 B).
   Discussion on the diet appears in the second book of the *Theonoston*. "*Seu De Vita
   Producenda, atque incolumitate corporis conservanda*," in *Hieronymi Cardani Mediolanensis
   Philosophi ac Medici celeberrimi "Operum"* Tomus secundus; quo continentur *Moralia
   quaedam et Physica* (Lugduni MDCLXIII), p. 376a.

given that we cannot live forever. And nearer to the end of his life, man is reduced no longer to eating but to drinking, with some difficulty, one egg yolk
a day, and to finish [life] through resolution, free of pain or illness. (108–9)

Even the smallest variation to the diet caused an imbalance in Cornaro, for which he risked going to his grave. We see it when he writes how,
giving in to the insistence of his physicians and family, he increased his
rations of food and wine to 14 and 16 ounces, respectively (86), and what
the consequences were to him when he was unable to drink wine during
the hottest months of summer:

every year from the beginning of July until the end of August, during these
two months, I cannot drink the wine, whether it is wine from some preferred grape or wine from some preferred region; for during that time,
wine, in addition to being completely contrary to and the enemy of my
taste, is harmful to my stomach. And so having lost my milk – wine really being milk for the old – and not having a way to drink, since waters that have
been altered and prepared cannot have the power of wine and do not benefit me, thus, having nothing to drink and with my stomach not well, I am
unable to eat except for very little. And this eating little without any wine
had reduced me by mid-August to a state of utmost fatal weakness. Capon
broth did not help me, nor did any other remedy. (118–19)

If that did happen to him every year, it makes us think he was not then
always as "perfectly healthy" as he claimed; but this is simply being clever
on our part.

There is a risk that the reader of the *Vita sobria* – fascinated and intrigued by the details of this most strange diet as described – may forget
that Cornaro only speaks about it as an example, rather, a point of reference for anyone who wishes to undertake the path of sobriety. But he was
always careful to advise that what may have been good for him cannot
work for everyone, and that each person, being the perfect physician to
himself, can find a suitable and effective diet:

those with a good [[complexion]]* can eat many other kinds and qualities
of food, and in greater quantity, and likewise drink wine; so that although
his life is a sober one it will not therefore be a restricted life as is mine, but
more open. (121)

---

* [Double square brackets indicate insertions placed by Milani.]

The lesson of Cornaro is one of an absolute simplicity:

> This [[sober]] life only consists of the following two things: quantity and
> quality. The first, quality, simply consists of not eating foods or drinking
> wines contrary to one's stomach; quantity consists of not eating or drinking
> except the amount the stomach can easily digest. That quantity and that
> quality, however, should be understood by the time a man reaches forty,
> fifty, or sixty years of age, and whoever maintains these two orders, lives an
> ordered and sober life, which has so much virtue and power that within
> that body the humours are perfected, balanced and integrated. Thus made
> good, the humours cannot be activated nor altered by any other disorders
> the body may have – suffering the cold and heat, being over tired, fasting,
> and others – if they are not too extreme. (109–10)

Cornaro continuously returns to the twin concepts of *quantity* and *quality*:

> the food I always ate and the wine I drank – being those suitable to my
> complexion and of suitable quantity – in the same way they left their virtue
> in my body, so too they left [my body] without difficulty, not having first
> generated within me any bad humour. (82)

Even proverbs are brought into discussion, and he asserts that the proverb stating "what tastes good nourishes and is beneficial" is completely
false, whereas two others are "natural and the most true":

> the one that says, whoever wishes to eat a lot need eat a little, which is said
> only because eating little leads to a long life, and living long leads to eating
> a lot; and the other, that the food left uneaten is more beneficial, because
> after eating, what has already been eaten is of no benefit. (85–6)

The rule of quantity and of quality is not an invention of Cornaro. It
goes back to Galen, [with whose work] besides, Cornaro proves to be
quite familiar; but the physician of antiquity had only recommended it
for the elderly.[41] According to Galen, old age is "a dry temperament, and
cold of body, brought on with the multitude of years," and, therefore,

---

41 "The same respect, therefore, is to be shown for the quality, and the quantity of food,
because with every bit that the old exceed that limit, they feel great harm, whereas
the young scarcely feel it even if they were to make the gravest of errors. It is then
more assured to give a weak old man little food, three times a day, as Antiochus the
physician would do when feeding himself" ([Galen,] *Delli mezzi …*, p. 120v).

"something appropriate for the old" will be "that which, in fact, being in agreement with his temperament is good for him."[42] The body of the elderly, being cold and dry, will have to have an alimentation suitable to these humours. Galen advises:

> And as I likewise said of small birds, that the best were – having similar meat, as indeed many do – those living in the mountains, because the ones kept in cities locked up in cages for selling and fattened on liquids and plenty of food, are, in that case, completely contrary. The best meat for those who find themselves suffering in this way is partridge, and then the hens known as woodcocks, and starlings and blackbirds and thrushes. If such mountain birds cannot be gotten, then use the ones that live in the countryside – or wood pigeons – that stay high up in towers in various places around. Also good are the sparrows that make their nests on roofs and towers. And they prefer these towers high up in steep locations. And hens that are kept here on the ground in the courtyard will be just as good. Old people who are thus indisposed are forbidden from having the milk of any animal other than that of the ass – for its being lighter than all others.[43]

We see that the alimentary prescriptions of Galen are very similar to those that Cornaro adopts; but what surprises is the extraordinary work of reducing to the simple elementary rule of *quantity-quality* that Cornaro succeeded in making out of the teachings of the classical maestro. It is sufficient to compare it to a passage by Marsilio Ficino that also goes back to Galen:

> But to return to our account: meat which is rather moist is not approved (...) nor that which is hard or dry as that of hares or beef-cattle that have gotten too old, but a moderate sort of meat is approved, as that of barn-yard cocks, capons, peacocks, pheasants, partridges, perhaps even of young doves, especially if domesticated. Such also are young roebucks and bull-calves, yearling wethers and likewise wild boars. Nor do I reject the suckling kid and fresh cheese. I have indeed omitted small birds, for the frequent use of foods which are too fine is suitable only to the stomach which has no tolerance at all for denser food; but a healthier stomach acquires a fleeting smoke or moisture from these foods. Nevertheless, I do not omit hen eggs if the yolk is eaten together with the white; for indeed the yolk alone is

---

42 [Galen, *Delli mezzi …*,] p. 129 rv.
43 [Galen, *Delli mezzi …*,] p. 158 rv.

nourishment enough for weak men . . . . For indeed it is likely that certain long-lived animals contribute to longevity, provided, however, that one eats meat of this kind when one is young, and likewise, in turn, that other meat be sometimes roasted, sometimes boiled. ¶ There should be twice as much food as drink; the proportion of bread to drink should be two to one; of bread to eggs, one and one-half to one; of bread to meat three to one; and of bread to the moister fish, green vegetables, and fruits, four to one. The meal should not begin with drinking, nor should the drink be too abundant at any time. Something astringent and with no drink, or a small one, should always follow the meal . . . . You should take two meals during the nine hours of the day – both sparse, but dinner the sparser.[44]

According to Cornaro, however, diet alone is not enough to attain longevity; it must be accompanied by other simple strategies that regulate daily life:

other than the two orders mentioned above, which I have always followed in eating and drinking, and which are very important – that is, to eat only the amount my stomach can easily digest, and nothing that I know is unsuitable – I have also guarded against suffering the cold and heat, over-extending myself, interrupting my usual sleep, excessive coitus, remaining where the air is bad, and suffering either the wind or sun, which – also these – are powerful disorders . . .

As much as I was able, I have also guarded against those things from which we cannot easily defend ourselves; these are melancholy, hate, and other perturbations of the soul. (82–3)[45]

It appears clear that a sober life cannot be practised (verb) if not by the upper classes, but Cornaro is not of this mind and has at the ready a diet suitable also for the poor, as long as they are honest and, from what can be understood – workers:

And the old man, who out of poverty cannot get such foods, is able to conserve himself on bread, *panatella*, and eggs. And in truth, someone poor will

---

44 [*Three Books* ..., II: XIX, pages 181 and 183]; *Tre vite* ..., pp. 36r–7r.
45 Cf. Ficino, "The elderly should often refresh their spirits with herbs, chiefly with wine, and avoid either fasting, or waiting too long before eating or drinking, because when getting older, suffering hunger and thirst is very harmful to them. And having the same effect on them is fatigue of the body, and soul, and solitude, and melancholy" (*Tre vite* ..., p. 40r).

not be left wanting, unless he is a beggar, or what is called a beggar – but we must not think about that one, because he came to this [circumstance] out of his ineptitude and is better dead than alive, because he makes the world ugly. But if the poor cannot eat well on bread or *panatella* or eggs, they need only eat the quantity they can digest; and the one observing quantity and quality cannot die, unless from pure resolution without any illness. (114–15)[46]

Man has always sought to prolong his life and it is no surprise to us that Cornaro and numerous others before and after him tried in a thousand ways to achieve this objective. But in times such as ours, of preventative medicine and free medical assistance, it is difficult to imagine the enormous disparity then existing in this area, as well as between the poorer social classes of manual labourers, artisans, and small land owners and those of the nobles, prelates, and wealthy bourgeoisie. Only the latter could make use of the resources that the much criticized but powerful medical art offered. The "revolution" of the *Vita sobria* is precisely here: in making available to everyone, rich or poor, an identical medicine easy to use and, above all, absolutely free. The sober life does not require much expense; to the contrary, it is a source of considerable savings, something greatly appreciated by Cornaro, the fierce enemy of every unnecessary waste.[47] It is enough to glance at some prescriptions provided by physicians at the time to see that even the simplest ones – not to mention those of theriac or mithridates – due to the many and costly ingredients required, were certainly not affordable by everyone. But what for us is rather incredible is the presence, in many of the prescriptions, of precious gems, pearls, and especially of gold. In chapter XIX of the *Tre Vite* [*Three Books*] entitled "The Medicine of the Magi for Old People," Marsilio Ficino provides us with the following prescription:

Therefore all you old people, come here to the wise Magi who are bearing gifts for you too – gifts that are going to lengthen your life, gifts with which

---

46 Ficino had warned: [It will not be, therefore, unbeneficial nor in vain (…) to give some precepts for prolonging life to those of high intelligence, and each given to study: however, we would not want to have participate in this benefit, in any way, those who are indolent, or inactive, whose life can hardly be called a life] (*Tre vite* …, p. 40r).

47 A true manifesto against the wasteful ways of citizens and the clergy – including the cloistered – in the hands of Cornaro became the first oration of Ruzzante: Alvise Cornaro, "Orazione per il Cardinale Marco Cornaro" and "Pianto per la morte del Bembo," in *Due testi pavani inedite*, ed. M. Milani (Bologna: [Commissione per i Testi di Lingua], 1981).

they are said to have once worshipped the author of life. Come, old people,
I say, who are taking old age hard. Come, too, you who are just troubled by
the fear that old age is quickly approaching. Please receive gladly these gifts:
Take two ounces of frankincense, one of myrrh, again one-half dram of gold
formed into leaves; grind the three together, mingle them, mix them with a
golden wine to form pills, and perform this at the lucky hour when Diana enjoys the favorable aspect of Phoebus or of Jove. Thereafter take a small portion of this great treasure any day at dawn, and wash it down with a little drink
of wine – except if it be in the heat of summer, for then it is better to drink
rose-water. Moreover, if at any time any of you especially fears heat, let him
add a myrobalan, either chebule or emblic, equal to the combined weight
of the frankincense, myrrh, and gold. Beyond any question, this will guard
your natural moisture from putrefaction, this will ward off for a longer time
the resolution of the moisture, this will foment, confirm, and strengthen in
you the three spirits – natural, vital, and animal; again, this will quicken your
senses, it will sharpen your intelligence, it will conserve your memory.[*]

Cornaro nourished a profound contempt for those, who, through the
element of gold, sought an elixir for long life. With his total rejection
of alchemy, and his denial of any curative power attributable to potable
gold, he goes against one of the most followed and sought-after practices
of the times, if not by formal medicine then at least by a large number
of physicians and wealthy patients. We must not forget, on the other
hand, that Paracelsus in those same years wrote the treatise, *De vita longa*
[on long life], in which we find a true anthem to gold.[48] Alchemic practices, good only for making the rich spend their money and, as Cornaro
bitterly maintains, often to cause their death, are, however, outright

---

[*] [Kaske-Clark, *Three Books* ..., p. 231;] *Tre vite* ..., p. 61rv.

48 [Paracelsus:] "Ex universis elixiris summum ac potentissimum est aurum. De hoc
igitur principio tractabimus: Nam huius rationem si noveris, aliorumque quae a
corpore separantur noveris. Reliqua quae a corpore non separantur, infra ubi de vino
mentionem faciemus, indicabuntur. De elixiro igitur auri, quod ad praxin attinet, sic
habeto: Resolve aurum una cum omni substantia auri corrosivo, et idipsum tantisper,
dum fiat idem cum corrosivo. Neque interim abhorreat animus ab ista tractandi
ratione: Auto enim quatenus aurum est, corrosivum praestat, et citra corrosivum
mortuum est. Quare quintam essentiam auri, citra corrosivum inutilem esse asseri-
mus. Sequitur ergo, resolutionem denuo per putrefactionem esse removendam, et si
corrosivum tenacius etiam adhaereat: nam si tanta vis est, ut corpus servet, ac liberum
reddat ab omni aegretudine, neque id corrumpi sinat, quanto magis seipsum, idque
citra omnem infectionem? Corrigit enim, ac emendat quidquid non est syncerum.
Corrosivum igitur in auro nullo pacto corrosivum appellari debet: Vis enim arcani
superat omne venenum:

nonsense compared to other practices that are completely harmless for the patient but which stir within us a sense of horror and profound anger. Here then (and I ask the reader's indulgence for this lengthy citation) is what Ficino recommended to his readers:

Immediately after the age of seventy and sometimes after sixty-three, since the moisture has gradually dried up, the tree of the human body often decays. Then for the first time this human tree must be moistened by a human, youthful liquid in order that it may revive. Therefore choose a young girl who is healthy, beautiful, cheerful, and temperate, and when you are hungry and the Moon is waxing, suck her milk; immediately eat a little powder of sweet fennel properly mixed with sugar. The sugar will prevent the milk from curdling and putrefying in the stomach; and the fennel, since it is fine and a friend of milk, will spread the milk to the bodily parts. Careful physicians strive to cure those whom a long bout of hectic fever has consumed, with the liquid of human blood which has distilled at the fire in the practice of sublimation. What then prevents us from sometimes also refreshing by this drink those who have already been in a way consumed by old age? There is a common and ancient opinion that certain prophetic old women who are popularly called "screech-owls" suck the blood of infants as a means, insofar as they can, of growing young again. Why shouldn't our old people, namely those who have no [other] recourse, likewise suck the blood of a youth? – a youth, I say, who is willing, healthy, happy, and temperate, whose blood is of the best but perhaps too abundant. They will suck, therefore, like leeches, an ounce or two from a scarcely opened vein of the left arm; they will immediately take an equal amount of sugar and wine; they will do this when hungry and thirsty and when the Moon is waxing. If they have difficulty digesting raw blood, let it first be cooked together with sugar; or let it be mixed with sugar and moderately distilled over hot water and then drunk. (...) it is possible and indeed beneficial to drink blood, and that there is a power in human blood both to attract and, in turn, to follow human blood; and to reassure you that the blood of a youth drunk

---

Nam omne realgar moritur in elixiro auri, et in tincturam abit medicinae praestantem. Atque in hunc modum gignitur, aurum potabile post putrefactionem. Hanc dosim, seu mavis harmoniam quandam praescribit pervulgata Spagyrorum praxis. Postremo observabis de elixiro, cuicunque confertur elixir, idem ita trasmutat, ut haud dissimiliter sibi fixum porro maneat" (Medicorum ac philosophorum facile principis Theophrasti Paracelsi Eremitae *libri V de Vita longa, incognitorum rerum, & hucusque a nemine tractatarum refertissimi. Vna cum Commendatoria Valentij de Retijs, & Adami a Badestein, dedicatoria epistola, quibus Theophrasti singularis & excellens eruditio commendatur.* (Basileae, Apud Petrum Pernam, s.a. [[1562]]), pp. 58–60.

by an old person can be drawn to the veins and the bodily parts and can do
a lot of good there.[49]

It may very well be that such a vampirelike practice was a first attempt
toward modern-day transfusion, but to us the scene described above appears emblematic of the extreme exploitation of man over man.

I.3 The 1591 Edition and the Fortune of the *Vita Sobria*

Exactly twenty-five years after the death of Cornaro, in May 1566, the
"complete" edition of the writings on a sober life came out in Padua,
published by Paolo Meietto. Its editor, Evangelista Oriente, a Paduan
physician – friend and companion to Giacomo Alvise – declares in the
dedication to the new Pope Gregory XIV that the task to "organize and
emend" the texts was given to him by Giacomo Alvise, Cornaro's favourite grandson. The overall title of the work – in which the [sequential]
order of *Treatise, Compendium, Loving Exhortation,* and *Letter,* has been
restored – is *Discorsi della Vita Sobria del Sig. Luigi Cornaro. Ne' quali con
l'essempio di se stesso dimostra con quai mezi possa l'huomo conservarsi sano
insin'all'ultima vecchiezza* [discourses on the Sober Life by Messer Luigi
Cornaro. In which, using himself as an example, he demonstrates by
which means a man can conserve his health up to the oldest age]. With
this edition, the singular fortune of Cornaro's writings is born, since
all subsequent editions, up to the present [1983], are based upon this
one;[50] and it explains why the *Addition* had never been reprinted: even
Bartolomeo Gamba, the only one to return to the *principes,* followed the
indications of the *Discourses* in regard to the texts.[51]

---

49 *Tre vite …,* 1.II, ch. XI, "De l'uso del latte, e del sangue humano, per la sanità della
    vita," pp. 44r–45r. [◊ English translation:"On the Use of Human Milk and Blood for
    the Life of Old People," in Kaske-Clark, *Three Books …,* II: XI, pp. 197–9.] Cf. also
    Piero Camporesi, *Il pane selvaggio,* (Bologna: Mulino, 1980), ch. III [Camporesi, *Bread
    of Dreams …,* trans. David Gentilcore, 1989].

50 The dedicatory letter and the sonnets by Gualdo that followed it are found in the
    [*Scritti …,*] "Appendice." On the history of this edition, see M. Milani, "Appunti su
    Alvise Cornaro e la *Vita Sobria* in margine a una mostra a lui dedicate," in *Giornale
    Storico della letteratura Italian,* CLIX (1982), pp. 216–44.

51 The exception is the one edited by Bartolomeo Gamba in 1816 and reprinted in 1826
    and in 1830; the Venice one of 1848, however, simply plagiarizes the others. Gamba in
    any case did not compare the *principes* with the *Discorsi,* from which he took only the
    sonnets by Gualdo.

Considering that Giacomo Alvise was Cornaro's direct heir, he therefore must have had in his possession all of his grandfather's papers – as the Codex Vienna also proves[52] – and the absence of the *Addition* seems all the more suspect. At the start of our research, we simply thought that the loose sheet, on which the *Addition* had been printed, had gone missing, until, curious about Evangelista Oriente's allusion to "organize and emend," we gathered the texts of the *Discourses* together with those of the *principes* thereby discovering that [Oriente] had not limited himself to "modernizing" the writing and punctuation or to correcting a few errors by the printer, but had heavily censored the writings by eliminating entire passages from them.[53] Why? It is understandable that in full Counter-Reformist censorship, an image in which,

> surrounded by such beautiful children, I am then likened by whoever sees me to a God the Father, encircled as in paintings by His Angels and Archangels, (97)

all has a rather blasphemous tone and would be sensibly cut. It is odd to find, given the description of his grandchildren ("all most healthy, all most beautiful") – as Cornaro portrays them immediately before – that the "all most beautiful" would disappear (perhaps the children grew tending toward ugly); but above all it is inexplicable as to why passages from the *Treatise* and the *Compendium* in which Cornaro condemns alchemy, along with the lengthy final passage from the *Letter* on the death of the youths – would have been censored.

We have already stated how the early death of his two grandsons may have compelled Cornaro to revisit his own ideas and to admit that even the most sober of young people could die. In a subsequent reading of the two texts, the contradiction becomes even more striking when the reader is not fully cognizant of the facts that had influenced the author's rethinking. Giacomo Alvise, worrying about the good name of his grandfather, thus eliminates the passage in the *Letter*, doing away with the conspicuous inconsistency between the texts.[54]

---

52 For the Codex Vienna, see [*Scritti* …,] pp. 70–1. Also the Codex Marc. Ital., cl. xi, 90, containing the already cited oration that was reworked by Cornaro, belonged to the family of Giacomo Alvise.

53 In the text, we [e.g., Milani] have marked the censored passages with asterisks.

54 The reason for censoring became clear only after a connection was seen between the *Loving Exhortation* and the letters of condolences sent to Cornaro in July 1564 by Danese Cattaneo and Paolo Pino, in as much as the dates when his grandsons died had been previously ignored.

Censoring the passages on alchemy, instead, is entirely due to personal reasons on the part of his grandson. Let us briefly look at this strange story together.

In his *Inscrizioni veneziane* [Venetian inscriptions], [Emanuele] Cicogna cites – in regard to the brothers Giacomo Alvise and Marcantonio Cornaro Piscopia – several documents in which it is shown that in 1590 and 1591, the two brothers were involved in a massive scandal instigated by the alchemist Marco Bragadin known as Mamugnà.[55] The documents were also taken in part from the Codex Vienna along with the extensive correspondence exchanged in that period among the Cornaro brothers, Bragadin, the Duke of Bavaria, and his commercial envoy in Venice, Alessandro Crispo.

Cicogna relates this note dated 26 November 1590 (but the events are anterior):

Marco Bragadin, Cypriot, famous for knowing how to make gold, came to Venice where he proved it many times. He lived well in Cà Dandolo at the Giudecca. The news spread everywhere that in Venice there was someone who could make the finest gold out of silver; all the princes were therefore in complete awe, envying this Republic. He then went to the Duke of Bavaria in Munich, where he was decapitated: so setting off legal procedures against him throughout the world. Whereas in Venice, [Bragadin] was favoured and served by the first persons of that city.

Knowing the frequent trips Giacomo Alvise made to Cyprus – where the many possessions of his wife Caterina Bragadin's dowry were kept – one could presume that he himself had brought Mamugnà to Venice. But here it should be told that the Cornaro brothers were among the most avid supporters of Bragadin, and when the latter, with the backing of the duke's envoy, took refuge in Bavaria, they became the protectors of his family. In exchange, Bragadin managed to obtain from the duke – in the Cornaro's favour – a large contract for wheat from Bavaria to Venice. The Cornaro brothers had no reason to doubt Mamugnà, and the news of his sudden arrest was a real blow. Giacomo Alvise rushed to write to the duke in defence of his friend:

---

55 Emanuele Antonio Cicogna, *Delle inscrizioni veneziane* (Venice, 1853), VI, P. 1, p. 569ff. [On "Bragadino," also see *Sober ...*, p. 112n59.]

Most Serene Lordship: Since I entrust kindness to Your Highness, I am thus here to communicate to you that the execution we have heard to be by your order, against Bragadin, appears to me to have been prudent and necessary in order to remedy the grave malady of this abject sinner, who, blinded by the Devil, was about to fall body and soul, if, by the mercy of God, he had not been redeemed under the care of your Serene Highness, for whose singular prudence I see more acts of compassion yet to come. Hence, gladly proving to be that self same servant dedicated to you, I continue praying to the Lord for your prosperity. Padua, 10 April 1591. Your Most Devoted Servant Giacomo Alvise Cornero.[56]

A strange letter indeed and it does not lead the duke to reverse his decision. Instead, he advises Cornaro that Bragadin – having confessed his guilt – was condemned to death. Giacomo Alvise subsequently attempts to do whatever he can: he is still convinced that Mamugnà knows how to "extract gold," since he had seen it with his own eyes, and shrewdly counsels the duke not to rush things:

I am obliged to plead with you not to be rushed into so hasty a condemnation of death to him in that with time and with his life [spared] it could achieve what will be dearer to you than your country.

The plea, written 29 April, is to no avail: Bragadin had been executed three days before. The duke, to thwart any criticism, had sent on the same day as the execution a letter to Giacomo Alvise containing Bragadin's confession:

Today 25 April in the year 1591 at Munich

I, Marco Bragadino, having to go tomorrow before the Court of the Supreme Judge, do confess and do declare before the eyes of God that I have never known the way to derive the soul of gold, nor do I believe that anyone knows or is able to do it. But all that I have done was pure and simple deception, so too I say about the castings [in gold], and I disclose this to relieve my conscience. *Infra.* And continuing this path I went about deceiving those around me, when the Lord God took mercy upon me and granted

---

56 Copy of the Codex Vienna, fol. 132*r*. The text bears the information: "To His Serene Highness of Bavaria when he gave notice of having put Bragadin in prison."

me the grace to be discovered, so that I may pay with my life as an example
of one who offends the Highest Good, may He always be praised.[57]

The story, however, does not end here. The Cornaro brothers, sensing
that the duke has toyed with them, react by openly criticizing the killing
of Bragadin and mounting a true scandal. The duke's commercial envoy
hastens to acquit himself and assert to the Cornaro that he is unable in all
conscience to swear to [the credibility of] Bragadin: yes, they had shown
him a purse full of gold in their house but he had not weighed it and had
thought even less to test it. In the end, the duke finds himself compelled
to intervene with the full force of his authority and sends to the Cornaro
brothers an official letter in which he states that he need not answer to
anyone for the way in which he administers justice under his own roof:

> Etsi vero nobis summopere curandum non est, quid quisque de nostris ac-
> tionibus sentiat, dum conscientia nobis testis sit, et leges, nos aequitatem
> coluisse, penitusque servasse: cum tamen iis sermonibus, quos sparsisse vos
> dicunt, nostra aliquo modo commacularetur dignitas, et avita laus iustitiae,
> quam tutari volumus et debemus.[58]

Cornaro's favourite grandson not only is an ardent supporter of alchemy but a recognized, even if unfortunate, alchemist. This is briefly
shown in the correspondence found in the Codex Vienna. It is only reasonable, therefore, that to protect his own good name, he would in this
case censor the passages in which his inflexible grandfather condemns
the ancient science and its followers.

As to the *Addition*, the point from which we departed, there is now no
doubt that its exclusion was owing to a deliberate act of censorship by his
grandson, attributable to Counter-Reformist murmurings, given the arguments of a theological nature that Cornaro touches upon in his writing.

---

57 Codex Vienna, fol. 131r. The text of the letter, which here appears to be damaged in
    some places, was combined with that of the Codex Correr reported by Cicogna
    (p. 570); which, however, presents some variations.

58 Codex Vienna, fol. 138r: [Latin translation: Although we do not care too greatly about
    what a person hears concerning our actions – as long as our conscience, and the law,
    bears testament that we took care of justice, overseen in a thorough way – however,
    with these utterances, which they say you circulate, in this manner our dignity could
    be poisoned and our ancestral renown for fairness, which we will and must protect].
    On this matter, which involved various personalities in Padua and Venice, we shall
    return with a work currently in preparation. [Prof Ivano Paccagnella advises that
    unfortunately this work was not completed.]

The *Discorsi* immediately won a good number of readers, many of whom, convinced by the example of Cornaro, became dogged followers of the sober life. The Flemish Jesuit, Leendert Leys, better known as Leonardus Lessius, wrote a treatise on the matter himself under the promising title *Hygiasticon, seu Vera ratio valetudinis bonae et vitae una cum sensuum, indicii, et memoriae integritate ad extremam senectutem conservandae* [*Hygiasticon* or the right course in preserving health and life into extreme old age], published in Antwerp in 1613. It had great success and was reprinted many times even if the author, who died just before reaching seventy years, did not represent himself as an example of great longevity; but to his own text, the theologian had attached the Latin translation of Cornaro's first *Discorso,* as a result of which it was made known to most of the European public.[59]

The first translations were based on the Lessius version [in Latin]: the one by the English poet George Herbert appeared posthumously at Cambridge in 1634 (but it had already circulated for some time in manuscript form), and the French one by Sébastien Hardy in 1646, which was followed a year later by the three other *Discorsi.* Editions from the second half of that century consisted of complete translations that were often accompanied by writings and opinions on Cornaro and his work, following the example of the French editions.

The history of Cornaro's work in translation is particularly interesting for what it says about the circulation of ideas in centuries past, not only in Europe, albeit not easy to track. In regard to the success of the *Discourses* in the English-speaking world, the reader is directed to what we have said in another work;[60] as for other versions, we limit ourselves to indicating those known up to the present [1983] in the list.* We will note here only a few curiosities: the Russian translation appeared shortly after the Polish one, completed under the reign of Catherine the Great

---

59 *Hygiasticon, seu Vera Ratio Valetudinis Bonae et Vitae una cum Sensuum, Indicii, & Memoriae integritate ad extremam senectutem conservandae: Auctore Leonardo LESSIO, Societas Iesu Theologo. Subiungitur Tractatus Ludovici CORNARI Veneti, eodem pertinens, ex Italico in Latinum sermonem ab ipso Lessio translatus* (Antuerpiae, Ex Officina Plantiniana, Apud Viduam & Filios Io. Moreti, MDCXIII). Subsequent editions were those at Antwerp 1614, Milan 1615, and Venice 1617; and several others thereafter up to the [nineteenth century] together with translations in several European languages. Lessio was born in Brecht in 1554, and died in Leuven in 1623. His translation consists of the entire first "Discourse" – that is, the *Treatise* – to which he joins the passage from the *Loving Exhortation* regarding the monks.

60 Milani, "Come raggiungere …," [Milani, "Immortality …," in *Sober* …, p. 183.]

* [The list, not included here, is found in the Italian edition, *Scritti* …, pp. 68–9.]

in the year in which Russian armies were occupying Poland. But to find
the first translation in Castilian, we must go to Lima in 1694, where it had
been published at the express desire of the Viceroy and Captain General
of Peru, Count de la Monclova.[61]

As to the number of translations and respective editions in various
countries, its computation proves to be hopeless, if not impossible. Let
us recall, by way of example, that in Great Britain more than one hundred editions were printed over the course of three centuries, but the
number of translators was only four: two in the 1600s, who, however,
relied on the one by Lessius; and two in the 1700s. Of these last two, only
one had translated directly from the original, even publishing the Italian
text (the Venice edition of 1620); the other was cleverly reprised from a
French translation of 1701.

Finally worthy of mention is a curious Latin translation that Bernardino
Ramazzini published in Padua in 1714 embellished with detailed medical notes. Ramazzini publishes the Lessius version, to avoid, as he explains, being accused of plagiarism and he adds his own translation of
the *Lettera al Patriarca* [*Letter to the Patriarch*] taken from the *Discourses*.[62]

In Italy, all editions of the *Vita sobria* issued between 1616 and 1970 –
apart from the one by Gamba and the one in Venice in 1848 – are
simple revivals of the text from the *Discourses*, given that reprints of
the edition immediately preceding it are ongoing, to which a slight
retouching of punctuation and spelling is occasionally done. In the
1800s, the *Discourses* began to be published along with other short
"moral" writings, such as the discourse to youth by Silvio Pellico, or
the treatise on family by Pandolfini, other than, of course, the one by
Lessius in translation. Even the edition edited by Pompeo Molmenti
in 1905 does not differ from those preceding it, and in regard to the

---

61 The Peruvian edition seems to be the first in the Spanish language, cf. Antonio Palau
    y Dulcet, *Manual de librero hispanoamericano*, Barcelona 1951, *s.v.*

62 *Annotationes in librum Ludovici Cornelii De Vitae Sobriae Commodis Bernardini Ramazzini*
    Practicae Medicinae in Patavino Gymnasio Professoris Primarii Serenissimo Principi
    Clementi Joanni Federico Estensi dicatae (Patavii MDCCXIV, Ex Typographia Jo:
    Baptistae Conzatti). Ramazzini does not explain why he added only the "Letter"
    and not the other *Discourses* as well. Perhaps he felt they were too repetitive and that
    Lessio's text was adequate to his purpose: "Contentus itaque esse volui, ut solum hunc
    Tractatum commentariis, seu annotationibus physicis, phylologicis, prout tulit occasio
    adornarem, cui negotio tempus vacationum a publicis lectionibus huius anni succisivis
    horis impendi."

information about Cornaro's life that the historian provides in his introduction, it is taken from the essay by Emilio Lovarini *Le ville edificate da Alvise Cornaro* [buildings constructed by A. C.] published in 1899.[63] The text by Molmenti was revived by [Augusto] Castaldo in 1911, by [Pietro] Pancrazi in 1938, by [Giuseppe] Fiocco in 1965, and by [Arnaldo] Di Benedetto in 1970.

The work by Lovarini, who rediscovered Beolco [Ruzzante] and his patron, ignited an entire series of studies on Ruzzante and Cornaro, from the ones by [Alfredo] Mortier to those fundamental by Giuseppe Fiocco, Paolo Sambin, Emilio Menegazzo, Ludovico Zorzi, and Giorgio Padoan.

In September 1980, the exhibition at Padua dedicated to Cornaro – within the framework of the celebrations of [Andrea] Palladio – made known the Grand Old Man to a city that remained enthralled. Now it is finally possible to visit the Loggia and the Odeo, which for a long time had been left forgotten and in a state of total disrepair; while the excellent visitors' guide, edited by Maria Paola Petrobelli, details the two monuments.[64] The crowning of public recognition conferred to Cornaro, however, occurred several months later, when students from a newly built urban high school decided by an overwhelming majority to name their school after him.[*]

II Alvise Cornaro and His "Autobiography"

From the time that Emilio Menegazzo, after viewing the photographic reproduction of the funeral eulogy, had realized that it was an autograph, the text that for more than a century was held to be the work of

---

63 It appears that Molmenti had published the text on the wake of the success met, in Italy as well, by the American edition of 1903 by William F. Butler (*The Art of Living Long. A new improved English version of the Treatise of the Celebrated Venetian Centanarian Louis Cornaro. With essays by Joseph Addison, Lord Bacon, and Sir William Temple*, Milwaukee) from which it takes in part the title: *L'arte di vivere a lungo. Discorsi sulla vita sobria di Luigi Cornaro e Leonardo Lessio.* The American edition was reviewed by Vittorio Rossi ("L'arte di vivere a lungo") in *Fanfulla della domenica*, XXVI (1904), n. 11. The essay by Lovarini is found in "L'arte di vivere …," [ibid.], pp. 191–212. The more extensive study done by Molmenti, "Luigi Cornaro e la vita sobria," was published in *Curiosità di storia veneziana* (Bologna 1919).

64 *La Loggia e l'Odeo Cornaro a Padova*, edited by M.P. Petrobelli (Padua: [Canova] 1980).

 * [Liceo Scientifico Statale *Alvise Cornaro* (*Alvise Cornaro* State Scientific Highschool) in Padua, Italy.]

[the grandson] Giacomo Alvise suddenly lost all biographical authority and became a text in regard to which it was wiser to be diffident.[65] The scholar was ready to deny the validity of Cornaro's words after having discovered that they stated an age progressively greater than was his actual age; as a consequence, everything he recounted about himself could be misleading or exaggerated, if not in fact entirely fabricated.[66]

The eulogy, together with the letter in which his grandson relates the last days of his grandfather's life, was published by Cicogna in the *Inscrizioni* as a "long letter by the same Giacomo Alvise to his same compatriot, in which he recounts the last moments of his old grandfather, his virtues, and lists his works." Cicogna offers the transcription according to a "most exact" copy that "the kind and illustrious man Enrico Cornet (…) took from Giacomo Alvise's autograph" already existing in the Codex Vienna.[67] All subsequent editions of the eulogy were to reproduce the one provided by Cicogna, which, with respect to the original, is anything but the "most exact" as was later shown by Mortier; yet, not immune from misrepresentation and error is the one by Menegazzo, who had a microfilm of the codex. On the other hand, Cornaro's handwriting – sinewy and written with the tip of the nib – in the "outlines" found in the Codex Vienna is particularly tight and very minute, with cancellations and corrections that often render its reading quite arduous.

---

65 [Emilio] Menegazzo writes at the beginning of his important study "Alvise Cornaro: un veneziano del Cinquecento nella terraferma padovana," in *Storia della Cultura Veneta. Dal primo Quattrocento al Concilio di Trento*, 3/11 (Vicenza 1980), pp. 513–18: "If one could draw without risk from autobiographies, it would be easy enough to trace a profile of the life and works of Alvise Cornaro. In fact, he not only speaks openly about himself in all his published writings (even in those of a scientific nature) during the course of his lengthy existence, but even, I believe unique to the history of literature, pre-arranges for his immediate survivors – and to be sure, thinking as well of future readers – an organic synthesis of all his human endeavours, giving to them the form of a funeral eulogy, which a friend or relative would have read or recited as something proper to the obsequies. I believe I have already demonstrated how much we should be suspicious of this self-eulogy." In fact, he had previously said: "What instead is unacceptable remains the fact that he had furnished – about himself, his work and his life – a version so tendentious and self-congratulatory as to surpass any flattering fantasy of a true professional funeral orator." "Tre scritti di Alvise Cornaro." Edizione con una nota introduttiva, in *Tra latino e volgare. Per Carlo Dionisotti*, II (Padua 1974), p. 601.
66 E. Menegazzo, "Altre osservazioni intorno alla vita e all'ambiente del Ruzante e di Alvise Cornaro," in *Italia Medioevale e Umanistica*, IX (1966), pp. 252–63.
67 Text of this "eulogy" is found on pp. 752–4 [of the codex]; the citation is on p. 696 of Tome VI.

Since no one had any reason to doubt the words of Cicogna – or rather, of his friend Cornet – scholars refer to this text by always attributing it to his grandson [Giacomo Alvise]. Alfredo Mortier, who gave a partial photographic reproduction, stated instead that it was not a letter, "but a funeral oration delivered on 8 May 1566 by Giacomo Alvise Cornaro for the obsequies of his grandfather."[68] No element exists that can verify with any certainty what the French scholar claimed, especially given what is said in the first part of the text – a kind of assertion that Cornaro later cancelled with a firm stroke of the pen – which cannot be a reference to his grandson but rather to a young protégé, identifiable, according to Paolo Sambin, as Orazio Lovato – the boy who in 1565 sang contralto in the chorus of the *Santo* [San Lorenzo Church].[69]

To us, it does seem strange that someone would think of writing his own funeral eulogy, but at a time when it was quite the norm to dictate one's own epigraph (recall the one by Speroni in the Duomo at Padua), it would not be cause for scandal. Not even the things that the eulogy recounts – allowing that it really was read – could have surprised the listeners, given that they were the same things Cornaro had repeated for years to friends and acquaintances, as evident in the letters published here in this volume. Furthermore, how could Cornaro, universally acclaimed and esteemed for his gravity, have permitted gross lies to be told at his funeral, precisely at the moment in which the very image of himself – on which he had been toiling for the past fifty years – would have found its highest confirmation? For a man who had modelled his life on an idea, who had constructed, step by step, his extraordinary longevity and who had boasted of having achieved every goal he had set for himself, I believe it would be unbearable for him to think that someone else could, upon his death, speak about him in a way he would not have wanted. Cornaro was a proud and reserved man, who loved wealth, "things" – and to the end regretted that the women in his life had stood in the way of his realizing an enormous reclamation project – yet, he did not love honours and hated "ceremonies," something truly very rare and not only for those times; still, by then, he was, for everyone, the "*Vita sobria*," and this was enough for him.

---

68 *Un dramaturge populaire de la Renaissance italienne. Ruzzante (1502–1542)*, (Paris 1925), I, p. 99n. Mortier seems not to have seen the codex but only photographs of this text. For corrections to the text by Cicogna, see [*Scritti …,*] p. 97n.

69 P. Sambin, "I testamenti …,"[in *Italia Medioevale …*, IX (1966)], pp. 339–41.

After all, even writing one's own eulogy is a modest thing; it is enough to read a few of the many funeral orations of the time to understand. For this work, Cornaro's style does not change: he is pleased with himself over the amount of success he has had in his long life, yet he speaks of it in a simple and direct manner without reaching for grand rhetorical effect, without flamboyant imagery. The vague impression we have of something almost out of sync comes from the fact that on this particular occasion its author cannot come down to a contingent reality. He does not speak, therefore, about his own age, makes no mention of the number of his grandchildren (important for dating many of his writings) and does not even mention his wife or daughter, who could have died in the meantime; the only one he does name is Ruzzante, at the time deceased some twenty years before. He does, however, commit the sin of describing his own death and for this he was not forgiven. And yet according to witnesses – even if he did not expire while singing "the devout prayer by Bembo" – his death, as he had many times foretold, was like the extinguishing of a candle.

Lovarini places the death of Cornaro at 8 May 1566, the day to which all other scholars adhered.[70] Instead, it seems probable that this was the date of the funeral, at least according to claims by the nun, the great-niece to Cornaro, in a letter that appears in a French translation of the *Discorsi*. The otherwise unidentified *petite-nièce* recounts:

> Il mourut à Padoue le 26 Avril 1566, et fut mis en terre le 8 Mai suivant. Sa femme mourut quelques années après lui.[71]

> [He died at Padua on 26 April 1566, and was interred the following 8th of May. His wife died several years after him.]

and speaks of learning of the news she offers directly from her father:

> Voilà tout ce que je puis dire de ces Centenaires, sur l'idée qui m'en reste pour en avoir ouï parler autrefois à feu mon père, à quelques amis de Louis

---

70 Emilio Lovarini in the essay "Per l'edizione critica del Ruzzante [1953]," in *Studi ...*, p. 128.

71 "Lettre d'une Religieuse de Padoue, Petite-Nièce de Louis Cornaro," in the appendix to *De la Sobriété et de ses avantages, ou Le vray moyen de se conserver dans une santé parfaite jusqu'à l'âge le plus avancé.* Traduction nouvelle de Lessius et de Cornaro, avec de notes par M.D.L.B. [M. de la Bonodière] (Paris: Coignard, 1701).

Cornaro, qui ayant vécu si long temps d'une manière si extraordinaire, mérite de ne pas mourir si-tôt dans la mémoire des hommes.

[This is all I can say about these Centenarians, what I recall from the times I spoke with my father about him, and to some friends of Louis Cornaro, who, having lived for so long in so extraordinary a manner, merits not to die so quickly in the memory of men.]

The date indicated by the great-niece is, on the other hand, contradicted by a much more reliable witness, that is, by Giacomo Alvise, who, at the end of April 1566, spoke of expecting his grandfather to die at any time.[72] What is of importance to us, in any case, is not to affix a definite date, but rather to observe how Cornaro succeeded in giving, by his own death, the ultimate confirmation of what he went on claiming for more than forty years. We see it in this account of his death by Anton Maria Graziani:

Ille paulo post abeuntem credo vitalem vim sentiens arcessi sacerdotes Jesuitas iussit, collocutusque cum iis de divinis rebus, cum se ante Christianis sacris rite procurasset, Crucifixi parvum simulacrum laeva manu tenens, laetum se, ac bona spe fretum venire, simulacrum intuens proclamavit. Eo deinde posito, decore sese in lectulo composuit, oculisque occlusis, tamquam obdormiturus leni efflatu animam egit, cum vix horae tres ab eo sermone, quem nobiscum habuerat, intercessissent.[73]

From which we can gather that Graziani did not personally witness his passing but learned of the details from members of the family who were present. Critics never gave much credence to Graziani's account, maintaining that he errs by one year on the date, in that he has Cornaro's death coincide with the nomination of Commendone – his patron – to cardinal. The error in the confusion of dates and circumstances can readily be explained owing to the late editing of the work; hence, to

---

72 Lettera I, *Appendice* I [in *Scritti …,*].

73 [See *Scritti …,*] *Appendice* [V] for the complete [Latin] text. [I believe, after awhile, feeling his vital strength abandoning him, he asked that the Jesuit priests come, and having conversed with them on divine matters – as when duly administering the last sacraments – he declared himself happy, and contemplating a small simulacrum of the crucifex in his left hand, he had faith he had come to his passage. And having put the image down, he gracefully placed himself in a small bed, and having closed his eyes, as if he were going to sleep, with a gentle sigh he surrendered his soul, though barely three hours had passed from the time he had that discussion with us.]

Graziani, it can only be imputed that he had Cornaro die at ninety-eight years, but such a "truth" had been upheld by the [Cornaro] family and was accepted by all his contemporaries.

Cornaro's age has been a torment to scholars, beginning with Cicogna, who, in discussing the letter by Giacomo Alvise, concludes thus:

> I have not seen the original [documents] of these letters, but if the date of 1566 (sixty-six) is correct, it is clear that Cornaro did not die in 1565 – since it was by trusting Graziani that historians say [so], and I myself have repeated – but admittedly in 1566. Which of the two contemporary witnesses then, Anton Maria Graziani or Giacomo Alvise Cornaro, should one believe, let others decide; I have said enough on it.[74]

It was, as we have said, Emilio Menegazzo to be the first to put order to Cornaro's tangled chronology, going so far as to indicate his date of birth as 1484.[75] We will not repeat here all the arguments made by Menegazzo, with whom we are for the most part in agreement; we will simply say that in adopting his method based upon a cross-check of the actual year of documents, the age declared by Cornaro and the number of his grandchildren, we are convinced that his date of birth should be changed to 1482. Leading us to that year are two texts: the first is the letter to the Magnificent Aluvise, dated 23 January 1551, in which Cornaro declares his age to be "70 in a few months," that is, of being 69 years old: therefore, 1551 minus 69 = 1482; the second is the will dated 23 January 1555, where he declares – precisely as in the preamble cancelled in the [letter] – to being 73 (1555 minus 73 = 1482). We recall that previously he had said he was 74 in a will dated 22 November 1552, 75 in the letter to Morosini (4 May 1554), and 76 in the letter to an unknown Cardinal (late 1554).

Furthermore, taking 1482 as the year of his birth, we see that the chronological indications of the eulogy perfectly match with the dates in the archive documents:

---

74 *Delle inscrizioni ...*, p. 696n. Remember that Cicogna maintained that also the eulogy was a letter by Giacomo Alvise. Cf. Patritium Gaugat, *Hierarchia Catholica Medii et Recentioris Aevi, sive Summorum Pontificum, S.R.E. Cardinalium, Ecclesiarum Antistitum Series, volumen tertium (1503–1591)*, Monasterii 1935, *s.v.* Cf. also [in *Scritti ...*,] Lettera XXXV.

75 E. Menegazzo, "Altre osservazioni ...," p. 260 and the table on p. 263; also see his *Alvise Cornaro ...*, pp. 514–15.

> By the age of twenty-two he decided to pursue his studies here in Padua –
> studying law to defend causes – where he remained for two years learning
> a great deal. (133)

The documents say exactly "iuris scolaris" in 1504 or 1505.[76] Still, we shall proceed with an order that is in keeping with [other] biographies.

Our Alvise, then, was born in Venice at the family residence – on San Bartolamio near the Rialto Bridge – to Antonio, the son of Giacomo and Angeliera Angelieri. He states that he was a descendant fourth-removed of Marco, Doge in the latter half of the 1300s, and specifically of the branch that, having settled in Morea, failed to see the importance of being registered among the nobles in their motherland. On the basis of this descendancy, Cornaro sought recognition of his own nobility from the Republic; but the request, which must not have been sufficiently justified, was denied to him. Cornaro, nevertheless, said he was always certain about his noble origins and wished to repeat this even at his own funeral.

Just like the Quarantia[*] in Venice, not even modern scholars accepted the story of lost nobility, rather, several accused Cornaro of megalomania; and yet there had to be some truth to it, because a likely story does not seem at all implausible for the times. Menegazzo thinks that "the temptation to insert himself into the genealogy of Cornaro patricians may have arisen (...) from knowing that among *his* ascendants as well there was a Rigo, a name that, from the patronymic, had then become a surname," (Rigo was the name of the Doge's son).[77] In reality, Alvise's grandfather, Giacomo, really was the son to a Rigo, who – if for reasons of chronology cannot possibly be the son of the Doge – could very well have been a direct [great] grandson. In fact, in postulating another Cornaro between the two Rigo, not only do we obtain a convincing genealogical tree, but we even lend credibility to what was claimed

---

76 Cf. E. Menegazzo, *Alvise Cornaro* ..., p. 514. Inexplicably the scholar subtracts two years from Cornaro's age: "in his self-eulogy he states having gone to Padua to study law at twenty years of age and of having remained until he was twenty-two."

 * [Quarantia: Council of Forty, official body of the Supreme Tribunal over legal matters within the Republic of Venice.]

77 In relation to this, Menegazzo, (*Alvise Cornaro* ..., pp. 517–18) brings forth much information taken from the testaments in the Cornaro family.

by our Alvise, who, on the other hand, must content himself with being a descendant not fourth but sixth-removed from the Doge.[78]

His mother, Angeliera, was the sister of Alvise Angelieri, the wealthy and powerful prior at the Collegio Pratense in Padua, upon whose inheritance Cornaro will later found his own wealth.[79]

At ten years of age, a boy "of superior intelligence and kind nature," Alvise was "given to letters, and by the age of 15 was quite well read." At around eighteen, he became part of the *Zardinieri* [Gardeners], one of the many *Compagnie di Calza* [stocking companies or gangs] which, at the time (it is the 1500s), revelled in the Venice Carnival. According to Cornaro, the "Giardinieri" were the first to recite actual comic plays with attendant musical intermissions. For this gang, he wrote theatrical pieces and composed music and songs. This fact, as well, was deemed totally false by scholars, since only young nobles could join the *Compagnia della Calza*,[80] but in Cornaro's favour we are now able to bring the passage from his letter to [Domenico] Morosini, in which he recalls that:

---

78 According to the genealogical tree reconstructed by Menegazzo in his cited study (p. 519n), between the death of Rigo the Doge's son, and that of Giacomo, a good one hundred years must have passed. Now since it is not probable that a son die a century after the death of his father (Giacomo died in 1460 and Rigo prior to 13 January 1368), in between the two there must have been at least one other Cornaro: which would explain why the son of this Unknown [relative] would be named after his uncle as the custom at the time warranted. Furthermore, if Alvise's descendancy really was fourth-removed, it should not have been very difficult for him to demonstrate his own nobility in spite of the adventurous story of uncles in far away Morea. And it should also be noted that the 85 years spent there by the Cornaro, more or less correspond to three generations. The family tree we propose is therefore the following: [MARCO, Doge (d. 13-Jan-1368), *father* of → RIGO (d. ante 13-Jan-1368), *father* of → TOMASO (alive in 1368) and of IGNOTO, *father* of → RIGO, *father* of → GIACOMO (d. 1460), *father* of → ALVISE and of ANTONIO (d. 1510), *father* of → GIACOMO (d. ante Nov. 1541) and of ALVISE "Vita sobria" (1482–1566), *father* of → CHIARA. For Milani's genealogy chart see *Scritti …*, p. 41].

79 On the complex figure of Alvise Angelieri, see Giuseppe Fiocco, *Alvise Cornaro, il suo tempo e le sue opere*, (Vicenza 1965), pp. 16–20; E. Menegazzo, "Ricerche intorno alla vita e all'ambiente del Ruzante e di Alvise Cornaro," in *Italia Medioevale e Umanistica*, VII (1964), pp. 182–91, and "Altre osservazioni …," [ibid.,] pp. 233–52.

80 Cf. E. Menegazzo, "[Altre] Osservazioni …," pp. 258–9. A fundamental study on the Venetian companies is by Lionello Venturi, "Le Compagnie della Calza (sec. XV–XVI)," in *Nuovo Archivio Veneto*, N. S. XVI (1908), pp. 161–221 and [*Nuovo Archivio Veneto*] XVII (1909), pp. 140–233; however, on the "Giardinieri," he relates only items taken from [Marin] Sanudo: "We do not know when the *Zardinieri* first arose; they appeared there for the first time on 16 February 1512. At the time there were about

all my companions from the Zardinieri company, who were many, are all dead and I am alive and I was the most mortal; one other was alive, that is, Messer Gasparo Contarini, said Vignati, but he died just days ago.[*]

Again, let us note that Cornaro's affiliation to this *Compagnia* sheds new light on the fact that Ruzzante often found himself in Venice to recite for the *Giardinieri* and *Ortolani* – [another *Calza* company] – as the omni-present [Marin] Sanudo records in his *Diarii* [Diaries].[81]

After the two years in Padua as a student, during which time he lived with his uncle Angelieri, becoming his active collaborator – if [in fact] he is the "magnificent little prior" about whom a student from the college remarked as having received a small sum[82] – Cornaro returns to Venice and sets up a practice as a defender of causes. He continued with this activity only for a few years because, upon the death of his uncle, circa 1511, he thought it more opportune to dedicate himself to developing the holdings that were bequeathed to him. A cancelled passage from his *Eulogy* confirms this:

the brother of his mother being dead, had neither sons nor grandchildren, [Cornaro] came to succeed his mother (?) for the posessions of this [uncle] that consisted of 200 fields of little use, because they were lowlands and for the most part marshlands full of canes.[**]

---

twenty-five [members], they wore a *calza bianca* [white stocking], elected Gasparo Contarini [master of ceremonies], and at Murano held festivities with a comedy, exhibits, dinner, farcical *momaria* [mummery], and danced until morning with twelve women from the countryside, though respectably dressed in silk." Other festivities took place 12 June 1514; on the following 8 October, with performances of the comic play *sbrichi veneziani* [e.g., Venetian rascals]; and in another comedy on 3 and 7 February 1515. The number of members had by then grown to forty-four. They were on friendly relations with the *Ortolani* [greengrocers], who invited them to dinner 15 February 1515. On 16 February 1520, they dined and watched a comedy, and at a party on 3 March 1522, always with his Lordship Gasparo Contarini, they requested that Ruzzante and Menato perform – (XVII, p. 159). Cf. also Maria Teresa Muraro, "La festa a Venezia e le sue manifestazioni rappresentative: le Compagnie della Calza e le *momarie*," in *Storia della Cultura Veneta. Dal primo Quattrocento al Concilio di Trento*, 3/III (Vicenza 1981), pp. 315–41.

  * [See *Scritti* ..., p. 160. Passage not included here in the Da Ponte edition.]

81 Cf. E. Lovarini, *Studi* ..., pp. 82–3, and Giorgio Padoan in the introduction to Angelo Beolco known as Ruzzante's *La Pastoral, la Prima Oratione, una lettera giocosa* (Padua: [Antenore,] 1978) pp. 18–20 and 26–7.

82 E. Menegazzo, *Alvise Cornaro* ..., p. 521n.

** [See *Scritti* ..., p. 130. Passage not included here in the Da Ponte edition.]

The Angelieri inheritance, however, was not limited to the marshlands of Codevigo, as would seem from the *Eulogy*, but included arable lands, fields, and woods, in addition to the house near the Santo with all its related active and passive perpetual land rights. If to this is counted the inheritance from his father (the residence at San Bartolamio) and the fact that Cornaro administered his own assets together with those of his brother Giacomo – always wih his full consent – including part of the residence in Venice, the 1,700 ducats endowed by their mother, the "hotel and commercial" complex at Portello, and the fields and houses in Este – one has an idea of the "goods" that Cornaro came to possess around the age of thirty.[83]

In 1517 at Udine, Alvise married Veronica Agugia da Spilimbergo, and the revenue from his wife's dowry brought new heft to the already substantial family patrimony.[84]

Having become a landowner, Cornaro wholly committed himself to agriculture, in which he saw a limitless source for high earnings and social affluence. With the objective of making use of his "fields of cane reeds," he did not hesitate in applying part of his "wealth" to the reclamation of them and – seeing that the sale of the "drained lands" provided income far superior to the necessary expense of acquiring them and to the work of reclamation – he bought another five hundred marshlands in Codevigo, and within two years had turned them into fertile fields. An immediate consequence was a considerable increase in income for the Cornaro household and an extraordinary improvement in the quality of life for the population of Codevigo that – with the elimination of the *mal aere* (bad air, but also malaria) – rapidly grew from forty souls to two thousand.[85]

---

83 See the first declaration by Alvise Cornaro on his heirs in [*Scritti* ...,] Appendice I.

84 Cf. P. Sambin, "I testamenti ...," [in *Italia Medioevale* ..., IX (1966)], pp. 300–1.

85 Scholars have always disputed these facts provided by Cornaro as proof of the benefit of "draining marshlands," and of his success as an expert agriculturalist. Menegazzo has recalled more than once that in 1507 the number of families in Codevigo may have been fifty, which could mean – figuring an average of five members per family – a minimum total of 250 people. And yet even this glaring stretch [of facts] by Cornaro does not at all minimize one basic truth – that of the extraordinary increase in population, which had occurred during his time; that is to say, in going from 40 to 250 people. The fact to be contested if anything is that final [number of] 2000, something that none of his contemporaries thought of doing, evidently because it corresponded to reality. In [1544] Cornaro had talked about 34 souls versus 650 (letter to the *Grand Commander*), in January 1551, of 1500 versus the original 40 (letter to the *Magn. Aluvise*), the number he repeated on 28 September 1556 in an official

The success achieved with his lands, good or bad as they were, quickly converted Alvise to the cult of agriculture:

> So I say that from early childhood I have always had a natural inclination toward agriculture, and, knowing it to be a just, sacred, and noble art, I undertook to work in it. And I do not regret it because by the Grace of God, through this art, I brought to my household much respectable wealth, as the major part of this art is to make unusable areas into the usable. Having some that were unusable, I had them reclaimed for cultivation, and purchasing others I did the same. Seeing this, several of my neighbours assumed me as a partner for a large quantity of swamplands, where in short order I showed them – contrary to common belief that thought them to be impracticable – how easy they are to drain, because I have drained a part of them, and another part will in the end soon be cleared. And in truth, the agriculture of reclamation is the true alchemy, which is the reason we see that all the great wealth of monasteries and certain private citizens has been made in this way, and not only do we see private individuals but cities become greater and powerful by this method.[86]

Sixteen years later in 1556, he will add:

> Nor is my goal in this in vain, nor founded upon the fallacy of alchemy, but on real and solid agriculture, which cannot fail, and the gains made by these means are the most just, most respectable and praised of all others and appropriate for gentlemen.[87]

---

document addressed to the Doge ("Aricordo de M. Alvise Corner, molto bello et utile alla conservation perpetua di questa alma città," in Giuseppe Fiocco, [*Alvise Cornaro e il suo tempo*, (Padua 1980)], p. 132 a). Would it be too risky to think that Cornaro might have switched the number of household members found in documents for that of the actual [number of] inhabitants? It should also be noted in Menegazzo that "in the Codevigo zone in 1514, Alvise possessed 25 [of them] between leasings and directly alloted properties: in 1544 and in 1562 these were 35. If we consider that in the "vicinity" of Codevigo there were, during the time of Angelieri (1507), about fifty households; and to the 35 alloted we add the 6 households from similar marshlands in 1544, and 9 in 1562, we can conclude that Cornaro was practically the sole owner of the whole village," (G. Fiocco, *Alvise Cornaro* ..., p. 537).

86 In the "Discorso de M. Alvise Corner da Padova delle provision della cavation della laguna, et accrescer l'intrada pubblica et della vittuaglia, apprensentato al Dominio dal detto," of 1540 (in G. Fiocco, [*Alvise Cornaro...*,] p. 102 ab). The writings we have cited by Cornaro are from the Fiocco edition, under advisement, however, that the texts were viewed in the original.

87 [G. Fiocco] "Aricordo" ..., [in *Alvise Cornaro* ...,] p. 126b.

At this point, his treatise on agriculture, which he was thinking about in 1551, must already have been finished for some time.

1517 marks a fundamental milestone in Cornaro's life: it is the year he married, as we have said, but it is also the one in which his illness began:

> Through the disorders he had acquired from hunting, and from other things such as suffering the cold, heat, fatigue, and so on, not knowing what continence was or a sober life, he fell ill at the age of thirty-five and remained so for five years, and neither the doctors' medicines nor bath cures could ever free him of this illness. (136)

Knowing Cornaro's ideas on "disorders," less than to the hunting parties and festivities that he pursued, we can attribute his illness more to the toll that the new responsibilities as landowner and land reclaimer had taken on a physique with a "poor complexion," as he himself always described it. His illness forced him into making a change to his life that was as drastic as it was abrupt. Perhaps it is the reason why we never find him alongside his great protégé Ruzzante in performances at the homes of Venetian nobles. But he made an exception on 15 August 1521, when together with Beolco [Ruzzante] he participated in the festivities for the arrival of the new Bishop of Padua, Cardinal Marco Cornaro.[88]

Alvise emerged from five years of illness (it is circa 1522) profoundly changed: the man once disordered and wholly devoted to the senses, became sober and continent and more determined than ever to follow the strict rules imposed upon him by the diet, certain of never becoming ill again and of attaining the ultimate goal of longevity. As for the rest, his life was as full and intense as before: he returned to hunting large animals in the woods around the delta and those in the Este Hills, and to theatrical and musical productions and parties; above all he returned

---

88 Cornaro's presence alongside Beolco is taken from a passage in *Prima Oratione* recited by Ruzzante at the villa at Barco di Altivole, near Asolo, to where the Cardinal had retreated after his long and taxing parish tour: "And so, along with my patron, I too had heard enough of the nattering they did there," Ruzzante says, refering to the lengthy official speeches of the Paduan scholars. A longer version of this visit is in the speech by Cornaro (A. Cornaro, *Orazione ...*, pp. 3–35). The familiarity between Beolco and Cornaro is verified in a document of 20 April 1521, which confirms [Cornaro's] identity as the *Paron* of the oration, cf. Paolo Sambin, "Briciole biografiche del Ruzante e del suo compagno d'arte Marco Aurelio Alvarotti (Menato)," in *Italia Medioevale ...*, IX (1966), pp. 268–70. Also cf. G. Padoan for what he has to say in the "Introduction" to A. Beolco, *La Pastoral ...*, p. 20ff.

to his work and businesses. Convinced of having before him at least another fifty years of life, sure of being able to count on numerous descendants – (the birth of Chiara, which occurred several years into the marriage, led him to believe he was still able to have many more children) – Cornaro begins to build also materially his own palace: his home already large and comfortable is extended with the subsequent acquisitions of neighbouring houses;[89] and in the expansive courtyard lying between the house and the orchards, the loggia begins to rise. It will be completed in 1524, as records the date carved into one of the capitals.[90]

Between 1522 and 1523, Cornaro was in Rome with [Giovanni Maria] Falconetto in search of ancient monuments for inspiration. By this time, the former painter had become the architect of choice for Cornaro, and together the two actively worked on plans for great new projects, among which were the restoration of the church in Codevigo and a manor – an actual and real villa so it seems – which description, however, no longer exists except for an eighteenth-century etching of the portal:[91]

a church once rather ugly that he made beautiful. So one could say that in that place he brought to God a temple, an altar, and the souls to adore Him; and he always took care of those souls with the two priests of letters

---

89 P. Sambin, "I testamenti …," [in *Italia Medioevale …*, IX (1966)], pp. 303–21.

90 The "signature" on the architrave, now barely legible, reads: *IO MARIA FALCONETVS ARCHITECTVS VERONENSIS*. On the use of the Loggia as a theatre setting, see the essay by Ludovico Zorzi, "Tra Ruzzante e Vitruvio," in the "Catalogue" to the Padua exhibit, [et al.], *Alvise Cornaro e il suo tempo,* (Padua 1980), pp. 94–104.

91 The bottom of the etching by G. A. Battisti bears the inscription: "Main entrance in the Ionic order connected to a building in a rustic order was erected by the architect [Giovanni.Maria] Falconetto in the year MDXXXVII in the Territory of Padua at the Villa of Codevigo in the district of the region of Piove with the aid of the most acclaimed [Messer] Luigi Cornaro, called 'Vita Sobria', now of the Noble Family Foscari." If the date is correct, the villa was built circa two years after the death of Falconetto. G. Fiocco considers the etching ([*Scritti …*,] fig. 43) to be the entrance to the church at Codevigo; cf. F. L. Maschietto, *Elena Lucrezia Cornaro Piscopia …*, p. 23n., who identifies the villa as the restored Erle house of today. For the other "constructions" by Cornaro, see the always informative essay by Lovarini and the studies by G. Fiocco, in addition to various essays in the "Catalogue" [*Alvise Cornaro e il suo tempo. A cura di Lionello Puppi (Padua 1980)]. The bridge at Codevigo, to which he refers in his "Eulogy," would be before 1540 (see the fine essay by Vincenzo Fontana, *Alvise Cornaro e la terra,* in that same "Catalogue," pp. 120–8), and we know from his grandson that Cornaro received an annual rent of 16 ducats from the city (P. Sambin, "I testamenti …,"[in *Italia Medioevale …*, IX (1966)], p. 343).

and music. He then made himself a comfortable and proper rural villa built according to architectural principles – so beautiful, so soundly built and so comfortable, it is unique to those surroundings – which he wanted to face with stone and so safeguard it against fire, war, and anything else. He had a number of dwellings built for the farmers, and a bridge made to cross the Brenta River, which flowed through the middle of that complex; work done not just by one man but as a communal effort. (134)

Cornaro's affluence spills over to the farm workers, who find in the reclaimed fields new opportunities for work. According to Cornaro, the cultivation of new lands cleared of marshes was the only way to escape the threat of famine accompanying the extraordinary increase in population that occurred at the beginning of the century.[92] He firmly believed he was an excellent patron to his workers, for whom he provided

---

92 [Cornaro writes:] "50 years ago in this city, there were not a 100 thousand men or, better said, souls, as we see from accounts and books, but now they have increased to 200 thousand in number, and thanks to Nature, in another 50 years they will be 400 thousand in number. And if now there is such great famine, we must make sure it will [later] fail [to be], all the more so because throughout Europe souls are increasing and the fields are rendering less. Because Time, which consumes all things, naturally goes on consuming the strength away from ground that has been cultivated and toiled. Farmers used to pay rent and they had wheat to live on, which they also sold; but now they do not collect any to pay their rent. If they want to live, they are forced to eat the feed their animals eat like ground sorghum and bran, from which the poor make their bread, and which cannot be good nourishment for them. They have thus lost the strength to work the land as they once did; similarly, their cows and horses no longer have strength, for they no longer have feed to eat. And this is all because the fields no longer render as they once did. Farmers are impoverished, their lands can no longer be worked and so we lack bread. This lack [of bread] together with the increase in souls has already forced many inhabitants to abandon the provinces and seek a living for themselves elsewhere, leaving behind country, home, and property, carrying their young children on their backs, suffering injury and discomfort and infinite misery" ("Scrittura in difesa del piano di bonifica, del 1565," see G. Fiocco, p. 139ab).

In 1548 the population of the land territories amounted to 1,590,040 souls. And that growth would continue despite the pestilence of 1555 and 1556, up to the great epidemic of 1576 to 1577: "In the ten years preceding Lepanto and the loss of Cyprus, the Republic made available a labour force with the highest contingent of labourers in central Northern Italy or in the most advanced economic area of the peninsula" (Daniele Beltrami, *Forze di lavoro e proprietà fondiarie nelle campagne venete dei secoli XVII e XVIII*, Venice-Rome 1961, pp. 1–2).

benevolent protection, similar in this to Diana's Priest toward the starving peasants in the *Dialogo facetissimo ...,* [dialogue most facetious ...,] by Ruzzante:

> I urge you to remain of good will, and do not fear the coming famine, because with the help of the goddess Diana, who does not abandon those who serve her as you do, I will provide you with the kinds of food you need, and be assured that these lands are reserved *solum* for you, and do not doubt that anyone but you may take any venison from here, which is as my sacred Goddess would wish.[93]

All is well then, if not for the fact that Cornaro continued to expand his own holdings by exploiting the wretched conditions of farm workers, like the husband and wife at Rosara who handed over two fields to him for ten ducats: it was their entire property and they sold them "volens sibi succurrere et subvenire in tam magna necessitate et extremitate victus, in tanta penuria qua nulla maior fuit unquam, ne fame pereant cum pauperrima familia."* It should be noted that the poor couple had received four-fifths of the amount stipulated in the contract and now had only fourteen *lire*.[94] This occurred on 4 June 1529. Cornaro had not even waited for the harvest:

---

93 "Dialogo Facetissimo et Ridiculosissimo de Ruzzante." Recitato a Fosson alla caccia l'anno della carestia. 1528. (In Vinegia, printed by Stephano di Alessi, 1555), batt. 134.

 * [The farmer, "wanting to help himself and bring relief to such a great and extreme need for food, which had never been as great before, so that they would not perish of hunger with the poorest of families."]

94 This is not the only example of usury reported by P. Sambin, *Altre testimonianze ...*: "There are countless leaseholders or artisans all from Rosara, except for one from Codevigo – the Counts from Collalto recently invested in almost all of the few arable fields, or those planted with food and trees, or valleylike – and who, almost all in debt to Cornaro and collapsing under the weight of their debts and needs, give up the *iura utilia et livellaria* of their land. The price varies from little more than one and a half ducats to 9 ducats per field and is doled out in two installments, one at the time of the contract – and this is almost always partially or totally swallowed up by previous debts of money or in '*rebus*' (millet, for example) – the other at the seller's request (usually during the summer – June, July, and into September)." See the letter by the Count of Collalto, which clearly shows the expansionist plan of Cornaro ([in *Scritti ...,*] p. 139).

 [Ducat = e.g., (approx.) two dollars, with a *lira* then being the smallest fraction of money.]

Zenaro, fevraro, marzo, avrille, mazo e an mezzo zugno al fromento. Poòh, a'no g'ariveron mè! Cancaro, mo l'è el longo anno, questo! A' sè che 'l pan muzza da nu, mi mo sì, pì che no fé mè le celleghe dal falchetto.

[January, February, March, April, May, and even half of June before the wheat. Blast, we'll never make it! Dammit this year is a long one! It is a fact that bread escapes us more than sparrows from a hawk.]

So opened Ruzzante's *Dialogo facetissimo*, performed in the year of the famine of 1528 at Fosson during Carnival.

In 1529, Cornaro becomes the sole administrator "of the income and property" of the Diocese of Padua, then overseen by Cardinal Francesco Pisani; a prestigious charge that will procure for him substantial earnings and not a little trouble, and which he will continue to manage until the end of 1537. The following year, on 11 February 1530, he enters into partnership with two old friends, Agostino Coletti and Francesco Forzatè, with the aim to "reclaim" several valleys around the territory of Calcinara near the Venice border. The earnings are foreseen as assured and the work not very demanding. Cornaro was in need of money to finance his "constructions" and "one of the finest gardens in the Este Hills, which is filled with various delicate fruits and the perfect grapes for making perfect wines" (134), finish the house in Padua, and make payments on his lease to the priests of the *Santo*, from whom, on 20 August 1535, he had rented a third of the large orchard behind the basilica from the road up to Pontecorvo across the river.[95]

The death of Falconetto (8 January 1535) does not interrupt the building plans of Cornaro, who instead decides to lend a hand to a new "construction" particularly suitable for music and, working from his own design, begins work on the Odeo.[96] From the Odeo, an underground passage emerged directly onto the orchards of the Santo. In the meantime,

---

95 Cornaro could enter the orchard by opening a door in front of his house, but he would have to have built a wall that went from the door to the river in order to clearly separate the part [allocated] to the priests. He could not construct anything beyond this.

96 According to Bresciani Alvarez, construction of the Odeo would have taken about ten years, from 1535 to 1544 or "[15]45, which however seems too long a time for such a man of action like Cornaro (Giulio Bresciani Alvarez, "Le fabbriche di Alvise Cornaro," in the "Catalogue," [*Alvise Cornaro e il suo tempo*, (Padua 1980)], pp. 48–55). In the same 'Catalogue," Wolters dates the Odeo back to 1530 (Wolfgang Wolters, "La decorazione interna della Loggia e dell'Odeo Cornaro," in the "Catalogue," pp. 72–9).

the main body of the house had been redone and decorated with stucco frescoes and sculptures. The outside façade was entirely covered in frescoes, the small chapel and stairway exhibited paintings by Falconetto, and "the heads painted on the ceiling of the bedroom, and the portraits on the headboard – after drawings by Raphael – were done by Dominico Venitiano."[97] The note of satisfaction that we sense in this passage from the *Eulogy* was thoroughly justified:

> here in Padua he then built the house we see, a kind not found in any other city. And being set in the most beautiful part he has surrounded it with six beautiful gardens of various forms – each adorned with different ornamentals – throughout which a wide and flowing river wends. In this house he built rooms that in winter remain warm without stoves or fireplaces, and in summer remain cool without ventilation or humidity. Having these beautiful and comfortable rooms, he lodged all the distinguished noblemen passing through this city, welcoming them into his spacious greenhouse with graciousness and unassuming courtesy. (135)

In the years from 1522 to 1540, the still sober life of Cornaro is crowned by continuing successes in all areas, but the moment in which it appeared to reach its culmination was on 1 July 1537, the day of Chiara's marriage to the young wealthy and noble Giovanni Cornaro Piscopia. Chiara, notwithstanding the hopes of her father, had remained an only child, and for Cornaro, who wanted numerous and noble descendants, there was no choice left to him but to find a son-in-law who was in a position to satisfy him on this account. Many suitors had asked for the hand of the young heiress, but they were all refused, until, beyond the horizon, appeared Piscopia, who, in addition to the qualities cited above, brought

---

97 From fol. 5r of the MS attributed to Marcantonio Michiel in the San Marco Library, we read: "In the house of M. Alvise Cornaro. The architecture of the loggia and walls in the courtyard, made of Nanto stone [Vicenza limestone] in the Ionic order is by Zuan Falconetto, the painter from Verona, who was a pupil of Mellozzo from Furli. In said courtyard of Nanto stone, the figures in the niches and the two of Victory above the archway were done by Zuan Padovan [Dentone], said to be from Milano, the pupil of Gobbo [Cristoforo Solari]. The Apollo made of Nanto stone in the first niche with the missing hand was done by the same. The small chapel and stairway were painted by said Falconetto. The painted heads on the ceiling of the bedroom, and the paintings on the bed, were done after the drawings of Raphael by Dominico Venitiano, [who was] instructed by Iulio Campagnuola. The fresco on the façade of the house was done by Gierolamo Padovano" (Codex Marc. It. cl. XI. 67 (= 7351)).

the most important and incomparable one of bearing the name Cornaro [of nobility]. Never was there a marriage more obviously arranged, but the betrothed were young, morally upright, and subject to authority. Chiara brought a dowry of 4,000 ducats, and to Fantino, the father of the groom, 500 ducats were paid "toward wardrobe expenses."[98] The marriage was celebrated at the Church of Santa Croce in the Giudecca with grand festivities, as recalls Cornelio Musso in a letter to Chiara:

> I know how well you have married, and how the many festivities honoured your almost royal nuptials, by the seas and by the lakes and all throughout the countryside and hills of that dear Padua.*

Husband and wife went to live in Padua in the Santo house under the watchful eye of Alvise. There, within sixteen years, Chiara presented her father with eleven grandchildren.[99]

The years between 1538 and 1544 were to mark – after many successes – a period of litigation and anxiety and family misfortune. Prior to this, there had been definite signs signalling the likelihood of what would happen, beginning with the initial differences existing between the reclamation partners and the Serenissima. In 1533, when the first embankments went up,

---

98 The wedding contract was published by F. L. Maschietto [*Elena Lucrezia Cornaro Piscopia ...,*] pp. 237–8). Cf. E. Menegazzo, *Alvise Cornaro ...,* p. 528. Of the many qualities of his son-in-law, he was, however, lacking in the one of good health, as learned from the first will of Cornaro (Nov. 1555): "I will leave to them [grandchildren] an ideal manager that I greatly value and respect, who is their father, a man of the highest intelligence and a perfect overseer (...) and though he is in poor health, which is a great contrary, yet being so intelligent and with order in his life he will conserve himself and being young will live for a long time," (P. Sambin, "I testamenti ...," [in *Italia Medioevale ...,* IX (1966)], pp. 355–6). Born in Venice on 17 December 1514, Giovanni died at Padua on 21 October 1559.

* [See *Scritti ...,* p. 242. Passage not included here in the Da Ponte edition.]

99 Their birth order is as follows: 1. Giacomo Alvise (13 September 1539 – 30 August 1608) at the end of 1561 marries Caterina Bragadin di Giovanni; 2. Fantino (2 September 1540 – early 1564); 3. Ferigo (15 November 1541 – July 1564), at the end of 1562 marries Elena, daughter of Sebastiano Venier; 4. Marcantonio (20 May 1543 – late 1590); 5. Isabella (1545 – 14 April 1609); 6. Elena (1547 – ?), marries Nicolò Contarini; 7. Stefano (17 November 1548 – Lepanto*); 8. Cornelia (1550 – ?), marries Girolamo Contarini; 9. Francesco (20 May 1551– Lepanto); 10. Girolamo (11 August 1552 – Lepanto); 11. Piero (20 March 1555 – 16 February 1639), marries Lucia Valier q. Piero. The present dates have been integrated with those taken from the [family] tree by F.L. Maschietto.*[Battle of Lepanto, 7 October 1571.]

an action was brought at that time to the learned Signory by a person, not
an expert in the field, who believed what many non-experts believe: that
[the embankment], a well-constructed part of the lagoon, could cause damage. The Signory wanted to go to the site together with experts to advise
them on the matter, and their findings were that the embankments could
not cause damage, and they did not want to proceed with that action. And
that this is true, Your Lordships can see by his office, where you find neither
a call for action nor even the minimum authority.[100]

In 1537, the sea flooded the lands that were being reclaimed and someone attributed the disaster to the embankments for impeding the out-
flow of water; but Cornaro defended himself by maintaining that, at the
time, the embankment dams were not yet closed, and that when closed
there was no longer any flooding. As a consequence, however, with the
umpteenth complaint filed "by non-expert and perhaps malicious persons," in November of 1541, the Signory intervened and ordered the
embankments to be brought down. The partners, one of whom was also
the attorney Marco Molino, immediately filed an appeal on the 23rd of
that same month with the writ cited above, but the Venice Magistrates –
strong as well in their expertise in the famous Cristoforo Sabbadino – did
not yield.[101] It is this the first lawsuit of which the *Eulogy* speaks:

> Seeing the number of his grandchildren increase, he decided to increase
> his property and acquired two thousand fields of marshes for draining, one
> quarter of which had been drained within two years. And all would have
> been drained if envy had not led to a problem, for it was argued that the
> drainage was damaging the lagoon, which, however, was untrue. (137)

Another lawsuit, yet more complicated and perilous, involved Cornaro
in those years. As the sole administrator (1529–33) of the diocese properties, and at a certain point also becoming a leaseholder (1534–37) – later,
only a leaseholder (1538–43) – he had a free hand, whether in managing
the ecclesiastical holdings or the improvements made, or even in the

---

100 "Scrittura in difesa degli argini in laguna," see G. Fiocco, [*Alvise Cornaro* …,], p. 120b.
   The "*persona inesperta*" can be none other than Cristoforo Sabbadino. [On Sabba-
   dino, see *Sober* …, p. 157n53.]
101 Cf. E. Menegazzo, *Alvise Cornaro* …, pp. 529–30. On Sabbadino and his opposition to
   Cornaro, see Salvatore Ciriacono, "Scrittori d'idraulica e politica delle acquae," in
   Storia della Cultura Veneta, pp. 505–12.

collection of rent and lease payments, and in the use of sums received. In exchange for administering the diocese, Cornaro had to pay the cardinal 7,000 ducats annually, quite a sizeable sum, which gives some indication as to what the earning potential was. For the rather complicated history of this lawsuit, we refer to the essay by Claudio Bellinati;[102] here, it will suffice to recall that Cornaro, in fact, twice risked going to prison because of his debts and that on 19 November he put the San Bartolamio residence up for sale in order to avert the threat of imprisonment. It is not known precisely when the real estate may have been sold, because Franceschina Petrucci – creditor in turn to the Cornaro brothers for 5,000 ducats – was opposed to the sale, though it must not have taken very long, since no mention is made of the Venice residence in the wills.

To the protracted and unpleasant dispute with the powerful Cardinal Pisani – who threatened to ruin not only [Cornaro's] fortune but also his good name – Cornaro traces the cause of his brother's death. For in Giacomo, having a good complexion but without maintaining a sober life, the "accidents of the spirit had their greatest power," and he was overcome "with melancholy humour, which is always plentiful in those bodies of an unregulated life, and it altered in manner and increased so much it made him die before his time."[103]

And yet the two lawsuits, the cause of so much worry and suffering, were always considered by Cornaro as having been won. He often speaks of them, emphasizing not only the final victory (in reality, we still do not know their outcome), but also the effect that they had in openly drawing attention to his strength of character, and in showing everyone that his success had not "come from good fortune," as many were alleging, but "dal suo inteleto" [from his intellect]. The passage from his letter to Speroni now becomes clearer and more significant:

> piles of money were taken from me in the matter of the Cardinal – true, against all reason much was taken from me – this however is not the reason I am sad. Rather, it made me happy, because if this injustice had not ensued, no one would have believed that – since I was good at making estate

---

102 Claudio Bellinati, "Alvise Cornaro governatore del Vescovado di Padova," in the "Catalogue" [*Alvise Cornaro e il suo tempo* (Padua 1980)], pp. 140–6. From this essay, with its wealth of unpublished information, we hope it will soon be followed by a more exhaustive and comprehensive work. Cf. also E. Menegazzo, *Alvise Cornaro ...*, pp. 551–5.

103 [Cf. *Sober ...*, p. 84]; Trattato [in *Scritti ...*,] p. 86. Giacomo, in fact, dies in 1541.

administrators and servants rich – I could have made a cardinal equally wealthy. Moreover, as you know, the officials regulating the waters caused me further notable damage, for which I assure you I am similarly happy, because I would not otherwise have become the liberator of our homeland, as I have become; because this injustice was the reason I found a way for conserving the lagoon, and hence, my homeland. Therefore, neither one nor the other of the above can disturb my happiness, rather, they have allowed everyone to see how strong and steadfast I am in the face of adversity, how astute and helpful and happy I am in good times. It is something I was judged to be the opposite, [something] considered almost impossible, since [according to others] I was always nothing if not most fortunate; yet despite this, I made it known that I could turn wretched fortune into good. (157)

With the turbulent and bitter years of lawsuits over, the nearly frenetic pace of Cornaro's prior activity appears to diminish markedly. Business dealings continue but are no longer as grandiose or risky: the "constructions," agriculture, and at that time the sober life above all was central to his thoughts. At his house, now completed with all its marvels, he lives quietly with his ever-growing family, talented protégés, and many friends, all of whom make up the "Cornaro circle":

And as soon as he would hear of someone with a fine intellect but owing to poverty was unable to demonstrate it – whether in letters, poetry, music, painting, architecture, or sculpture – he would take the person under his care and provide him with the encouragement and means for him to express it. (135)

At his home, he received illustrious guests such as Duke Guidobaldo d'Urbino, who, while there, met Tiziano Aspetti – called Minio – the artist for the Odeo stucco work.[104] The duke was accompanied on his visit by [Pietro] Aretino, who writes to Giovanni Cornaro: "I praise the hour and the point at which the Excellence [magnanimity] of his eminent Duke Guido Baldo deigned to bring me to lodge with him in the palace of your home."[105] Among the sculptors bound to Cornaro, the one who stands out, in addition to Minio, is Danese Cattaneo, whose beautiful bust of

---

104 On Minio, the artist in stucco, see Wolfgang Wolters, "Tiziano Minio als Stukkator im, *Odeo Cornaro* zu Padua. Ein Beitrag zu Tiziano Minio Frűhwerk Der Anteil des Giovanni Maria Falconetto," in *Pantheon* 21 (1963), pp. 222–30.

105 *Lettera* in *Appendice VI* 2, [in *Scritti ...,*] p. 263.

an old man at the Kunsthistorisches Museum at Vienna brings to mind, oddly enough, the portrait of Cornaro by Tintoretto. But to discuss the artists who worked for Cornaro or who came in contact with him would mean opening a long chapter on Venetian art of the Cinquecento, something that is beyond our competence, and on this we direct the reader to the essays found in the "Catalogue" to the [Cornaro] exhibit in Padua: suffice it to recall here the names of Andrea da Valle and Palladio.

It is equally impossible to offer in so short a space a complete picture of the men and ideas that in the "Cornaro circle" converged and circulated: from the young and the not-so-young "protégés" to the great friends, first among whom is [Pietro] Bembo, who was there in Padua during what were the happy years for Cornaro. On one side were Ruzzante, Falconetto, and Minio, and on the other, Tomitano, Speroni, Pierio Valeriano, and [Alessandro] Piccolomini – in a word, the *Infiammati* [Inflamed]* – and the many distinguished professors from the university at Padua. And alongside these were the agriculturalists, as Cornaro calls them, his partners in the reclamation undertaking, his attorneys and accountants, and so forth, up to the ever-faithful Girolamo Pelizon, about whom in his last will he finds extraordinary words of affection and recognition.[106] Among friends, the one to emerge in a preeminent

---

* Accademia degli Infiammati (the Inflamed) was a literary academic circle founded in Padua in 1540. Prominent members included Speroni Sperone, Benedetto Varchi, and Angelo Beolco. On this and other academies of the time, see for example Domenico Zanré's *Cultural Non-Conformity in Early Modern Florence* (Aldershot, UK: Ashgate, 2004).

106 [Cornaro writes:] "And because I love Gierolamo Pelizone [*sic*] so much, as if he were my own blood, and whom I raised, and who has served me as an administrator these many years, much to my advantage, managing my diocese property during the nine years that I had rented it, and he was most loyal in that endeavour; because there has never been anyone more loyal and loving to his patron. Therefore, I would like when I am gone, since this house will be left abandoned by my family – who will want to go where it is more practical and comfortable, by going to live in their own house in Venice – and so it will remain empty, in which case, my thought is that Gierolamo leave the duties he now has with Signore Pio de Ii Obici [Obizzi] and that he come to stay in this house to run it for as long as he lives; and that his expenses, and [money] for a servant and a farmer be paid by Giacomo Luigi, because the house will have to have someone there to live and run it. And should this Giacomo Luigi's ability [to pay] suffer an accident, being in Cyprus, and not being able then to provide for the above said expenses, in that case I would like them to be paid by my commissioners and heirs. And that in addition to the expenses appropriate to [Pelizone], and for a servant and a farmer, they will have to pay their salaries of

manner is the Franciscan, Cornelio Musso, who remained bound to the Cornaro family throughout his life; but to this great preacher, and other personages, we shall return later in the notes.[*]

Let us look briefly now at the *pavano*[**] aspect of the "Cornaro circle," that *ca' e massaria di Ruzanti* [home and estate of poets named the "Ruzanti"], over which Cornaro is the recognized *paron* [patron] and *massaro* [lord of the manor]. All scholars of Beolco, beginning with Lovarini, have shown how, following his death, the *pavano* tradition was to carry on with "minor" poets and authors, up until the appearance of the other great *boaro*[◊] Giovan Battista Maganza, called Magagnò. In this way, continuity was also owing to the fact that Beolco's fellow artists had remained united around Cornaro, as in the case of Menato or Marco Aurelio degli Alvarotti, the noble and wealthy landowner – and son of Cornaro's old friend Francesco – who was the Alvaroto that Alvise wished by his side in his private earthly paradise;[107] and so too in the case of Bilora, that is, Zaccaria Castegnola, who married Ruzzante's widow.

---

2 ducats a month, and that some money be spent so that he may dress well throughout the years, and have clothes made of linen and whatever he may require. But because things for Giacomo Luigi will go well, I know that he – who understands the value of said Gierolamo and his loyalty – will put him to work, for a few thousand ducats, by building a bread shop and other jobs. Moreover, by these means he will reduce his future expenses and every year he will make an acquisition that will be good for building" (P. Sambin, "I testamenti ...," [in *Italia Medioevale ...*, IX (1966)], p. 383).

[*]   [This reference applies only to Milani's edition in Italian: *Scritti ...*,]

[**] [*pavano* is a literary parodic language commingling the Paduan country dialect, devised by Ruzzante and others for their theatre pieces and poetry.]

◊   [*boaro*: from L. pastor boum: *bovaro* = *boaro*, the one who brings cattle to pasture, a herdsman. It is "a classical term which has social and linguistic connotations."]

107 A spokesman for Cornaro discusses the ones who may enter the new earthly paradise: "here we would like You [Lord] to let our *paron* enter with all his brigade – among them are also five boys who rightly make a paradise beautiful – and all his dearest relatives and so too his dear friends. And in that case we would like You to bring his brother back to life, and Foscar and Alvaroto and Ruzzante and Zacaroto and uncle Polo and Pacalonio and Moro and Pasin and Sirinzi; and all his many good companions, and all his hunters along with their good dogs that have died. And that the [Greghette] girls, the singers, be [notified] by mail sent immediately to Venice, for without them Paradise would not be complete. And after this brigade has passed inside we would like You to surround it with a fence and see to it that there inside the climate will be beautiful and fine, serene, clear, and always sunny, with no clouds or rain or snow or wind; and above all that there is no cold or heat but will forever be April" (A. Cornaro, *Orazione ...*, pp. 33–4).

Mo tutte le comierie e le canzon / ch'ha compondue Ruzante, in fede mia
/ che 'l le g'ha fatte apozò al so peon. / Sì, che 'l no fo el baston / an de la
so vecchiezza, e de Billora, / e de Menatto, che 'l s'in dise anchora?

[So that all the plays and songs that Ruzante composed, upon my faith
he did them leaning on his paeon. In fact, did he not turn them into
the cane for his old age, and for Bilora's, and Menato's – in what we still
recite?]*

So sings Magagnò in the sonnet dedicated to Cornaro.[108] Even within the
pavano patronage in which all the *boari* are poor and in need of protection, here Maganza portrays a reality based upon direct experience.

The Pavano Academy, which carries on with the older as well as other
younger intellectuals – such as the priest Giacomo Morello, known as
Morato, author of numerous rustic texts [villanelles] and likely commissioned by the *paron* to rework Ruzzante's third oration – will welcome, in
due course, new and promising poets. Among these is Claudio Forzatè –
contemporary and friend of Giacomo Alvise – who was a good *pavano*
poet also known as Sgareggio, and a worthy author of tragedies and rustic comedies.[109] Around Cornaro, therefore, the *pavani* continue composing and reciting and singing just as when Ruzzante was alive, in the
same way it had been done before him. Beolco, in fact, joined the group
that Cornaro had initially formed around himself during the years of his
disordered life, that is, before 1517: demonstrated by the fact that Ruzzante recalls in his *Dialogo facetissimo* several "good companions" by then

---

   * [This is one reading of the poem. Menato (*La Moscheta*) and Bilora (*Bilora*) are
personae from theatre pieces created by Ruzzante. My thanks go to Prof. Piermario
Vescovo (Università di Venezia, Ca' Foscari) for his kind assistance in interpreting
the *pavano* verses cited herein.]

108 See [in *Scritti …,*] the appendix for the text. Magagnò is part of the "group" of *boari*
from Vicenza, among whom it seems was also Count Marco Thiene, who wrote
under the name of Begotto; yet it is no coincidence that he would have Percacino
publish his first book of lyric poems.

109 *Delle Rime de Sgareggio Tandarelo da Calcinara in lingua rustica padoana* (Parte Prima,
in Padoa, Appresso Paulo Meieto, MDLXXXIII). The works in Italian are: *Rime del
Signor Claudio Forzatè* (in Padova, Appresso Giovanni Cantoni, 1585); *La Recinda trage-
dia di Claudio Forzatè. Dedicata al Clarissimo Sig. Marc' Antonio Cornaro fù del Clarissimo
Signor Giovanni* (in Padoua, Appresso Lorenzo Pasquati, MDXC), (the addressee
therefore is Cornaro's grandson); *Commedia pastorale*, unpublished MS, text in five
acts with intermezzos in Italian and *pavano*.

deceased for some time, who are the same ones Cornaro wishes to have brought back to life, still in their twenties, to be part of his paradise. With Beolco gone, the remaining "good companions" will change name and become the "*Ruzanti,*" but the leader will always be Cornaro; the *massaro* who will later compose and recite the lament for everyone in the *gran ca'* – the great house – on the death of Pietro Bembo. At the *pavano* academy, all the friends would somehow stay involved whether alive or dead, an example of this is found here in the epitaph that Domenico Lampietti – in art known as Lenzo Durello – dedicates to Tomitano:

Chialò ghe xe quell celente pavan, / Miedego in merdesina sì da ben, / Che de slettiere ha pin la panza e 'l sen. / El lome so è Bernardin Tumitan.[110]

[Who is that excellent pavano, a worthy doctor of merdecine, with belly and breast full of litters. Bernardino Tomitano is his name.]*

Cornaro's love for the theatre accompanied his love for music, and among his friends were many talented musicians, as we gather from Ruzzante's dialogue cited above. Like the spirit of Zaccarotto says in recounting the two paradises, the one for the contemplative and the other for the "good companions," of whom he was a part:

---

110 *Rime di Domenico Lampietti ditto Lenzo Durello. In lingua rustega padouana* (in Padoa, Appresso Paolo Meietti, MDXXCII), p. 37*v.* Tomitano died in 1576.

The "Pavano Academy" continues with the new *boari* – among them, Forzatè and Lampietti, under the patronage of Giacomo Alvise, and in close contact with the "Vicenza school" – into the next century. Participating in this during his sojourn in Padua is Galileo Galilei, friend of Giacomo Alvise – also because their houses were adjoining – and a great admirer of Ruzzante. He himself writes in dialect (in reality more Venetian than *pavano*); and one of his best pupils, the friar Girolamo Spinelli, under the name of Cecco di Ronchitti, composes the *Dialogo in perpuosito de la Stella Nuova,* printed by Tozzi in 1605, one year before the death of Giacomo Alvise. Cf. E. Lovarini, "Galileo interprete del Ruzzante" and "Galileo scrittore pavano?," in *Studi ...,* pp. 376–92 and 393–410.

* [The translation is one possible reading of this poem, since a play on words exists: for example, *merdesina* = *merde*cine = medicine (Tomitano was a physician). Piermario Vescovo (Università di Venezia) suggests that doctor of "merdesina" (*merda* = shit) possibly refers to what a doctor would in fact have to examine from a patient. Here the "s" in *slettiere* is prosthetic, for euphonic effect, hence the term *s-lettiere* is *lettiere,* pl., which can mean "litters," denoting either the material (e.g., straw or leaves) to absorb waste (*merda*), or the stretchers to carry (or to bed) patients who are sick or wounded. Tomitano, close friend of Cornaro, was also a learned scholar and author, so *s-lettiere* also plays upon *lettere* or "letters" = erudition, learning.]

Hieronimo Scrinzi did not come to him. We hear the beautiful sound of his horn so well when we want to go hunting but we do not see him.*

And he adds:

Uncle Paolo is here and more pleasant than ever, completely revitalized. I have only now left him, he was with Alessandro Pacalono, who was [encouraging] him with the sound of his lute, as well as many other good friends, there where it was the greatest place with the greatest laughter in the world.**

We know from Cornaro himself that Ruzzante was an exceptional author and composer of songs, and a long reworked passage of [Cornaro's] oration is dedicated to the art of two singers from Venice, the Greghette sisters, who were also remembered together with Ruzzante in the letter to the Magnificent Aluvise:

enjoying (...) so fine a number of grandchildren, who now entertain me with the divine music of the Signore Greghette, who wanted [my grandchildren] as their only heirs, in addition to their still being heirs to the great Ruzzante.◊

He will subsequently write to Morosini:

my rooms are built according to reason, where music that is not good sounds good and angelic and [where my grandchildren], having angelic voices as well as their faces, sing angelically. And as my voice is better than ever, I sing surrounded by them, and for whoever sees or hears me, I am likened to God the Father among Angels or Archangels. And with this music and in this paradise I take my leave.♦

In his letters, Cornaro loved to talk about these musical *intertenimenti* [entertainments], and his words are repeated in Mario Savorgnan's response:

---

  * [*Scritti* ..., p. 56.]
  ** [*Scritti* ..., p. 56.]
  ◊ [*Scritti* ..., p. 152.]
  ♦ [*Scritti* ..., pp. 160–1.]

to teach others (…) to make as if by their own hands a buoyant atmosphere and eternal spring, and finally a Paradise filled with an order of angels, with that sweetest and gentlest of goodwill and accord we could ever hope to hear if not in Heaven when not so very good music is made excellent, and the notes made better with one voice answering the other in clear splendid harmony.*

We do not have a way to identify which musical genre may have been performed at Cornaro's house, but no doubt, along with the traditional, the latest trends were being played: from the *villotta* to the *frottola* to the madrigal, from the simplicity of popular trends to the refinement of the chromatic, with which the Venetian school was then experimenting. Cornaro sang while accompanying himself on the lute and he was rather proud of his own voice, which was still strong and melodious, despite his age. He speaks of it in all his writings on the sober life and in various letters. A year before his death, at 83 years, he remarks in the *Loving Exhortation*:

and my voice, which before tended to be lower, is stronger and has become melodious, for which I am now obliged to sing my morning and evening prayers in a strong voice, whereas once I spoke them in a subdued and low one. (126)

In his letter to Cardinal Pisani in June of 1565, he adds:

Nor in any part [of me] are my senses diminished whether in my memory or intellect, not even my voice, which is the first thing one loses, because I sing my prayers in a more or less strong voice, [which] as I told you was once subdued and low.**

He was already certain in 1563 that he would have died singing his own prayers (121), and in his *Eulogy* states this as fact, something that in reality did not come to pass, as we learn from his grandson's letter: "Though his tongue is quite swollen, his brain works" (181).

Among the musicians who frequented his home was also a young woman, Petrinella da Armer di Candia, who for several years was

---

* [*Scritti* …, pp. 198–9.]
** [*Scritti* …, p. 230.]

Cornaro's mistress. He speaks of her in the autograph draft of his first will with the aim to disavow paternity of her child, Cornelia, whom he had recognized in a previous bequest:

> And because Madonna Petrinella da Amer di Candia said that her daughter Cornelia is my daughter, which she is not, given that Messer Iacopo Fuschari, Messer Agostin Coleti and Messer Bernardino knew that this Madonna Petrinella was hoping to have a child by me during the past three years, which she did not succeed in doing. In order to have a child, she became infatuated with Messer Zordan Coleti, who worked there as a servant in the house and by him remained with child. And that this is seen in his likeness of said Cornelia, he cannot deny that she is his daughter, because there is nothing of me in her. Once we discovered she was pregnant by the aforementioned, he confessed to being infatuated with her, and she has still not denied it, so it is clear she is not my daughter.[111]

To be then free of the inconvenience of having a mistress around, Cornaro convinced her to leave for Rome, where she could better develop her talent, promising that he would pay for all her expenses, including a return trip in the event that she was unsuccessful. Things, instead, went extremely well for Petrinella, who quickly became wealthy, "but she did not know how to manage it, because she became involved with a Roman lad and wanted him for a husband, which is why the youth's father made him hold on to her, and after he had squandered [her money] and she understood the danger, she escaped from Rome and returned to Venice." Cornaro declares that, given the circumstances, he is no longer obliged to maintain his promise; nevertheless, for the benefit of Petrinella, he arranges a lifetime inheritance of ten ducats a year. His natural daughter, denied in the first will, is however recognized in the last one; but [Cornelia] does not receive any inheritance from [Cornaro] her father, because he had arranged her marriage, "by then some years ago, with a suitable dowry, to Messer Aluvise de Lazera, the lawyer who earns

---

111 [Paolo] Sambin, "I testamenti ...," [in *Italia Medioevale* ..., IX (1966)], p. 360ff. Petrinella could be one of the two Greghette singers who Cornaro extolled in his writings, but whom he does not name after 1551. The matter, related in great detail in his will (November 1552), must have recently occurred, which would confirm the identification proposed by us. Cf. what was already said in A. Cornaro, *Orazione* ..., p. 17ff.

a thousand ducats a year and by her has just the one little girl, who will be the heir to her beloved Madona Caterina, who has some means."[112]

Even Cornaro, then – and in the midst of an entirely sober life – had extra conjugal adventures that had cost him quite a sum of ducats. In the end, everything must have been satisfactorily resolved, which is why perhaps in the notarized draft of his first will he omits the story of Petrinella and Cornelia and inserts there instead the passage relative to Bishop Musso.

Cornaro decided to make a will subsequent to his decline resulting from the first illness that had kept him so ill throughout the entire winter of 1552–1553. Another illness will strike him the following winter, but nothing [in his will] was changed in respect to the year before and he does not go back to it. Instead, he draws up another will in January 1555, after a new addition to the family: the birth of an eleventh grandchild, occurring almost three years after the last – (remember, Chiara's reproductive average is one child per year) – leads him to hope that the same rhythm would return and that the number of his descendants would grow; he thus sees himself compelled to reduce substantially the amounts bequeathed to his servants.[113] Moreover, he had by then decided to go ahead with considerable changes to the layout of the inner courtyard, moving the stalls towards the hen-house and building in their place a portico that will echo that of the Odeo, and then connect the old residence by constructing two other arcades to match the existing ones

---

112 To Cornelia, he had given 1000 ducats as a dowry against the 15 thousand designated for his grandchildren. P. Sambin, (["I testament …," in *Italia Medioevale* …, IX (1966)], p. 303) speaks of two distinct natural daughters, in that the second Cornelia would be the daughter of Caterina. But here, "madona" signifies "mother-in-law," making Caterina the mother of the husband. Born a few years before 1552 (the little girl is [by then] big enough to show "in her looks" traits of the father), Cornelia could very well have been already married and the mother of "a little girl" in April 1565. As to Alvise da Lazera, it could be a reference to the Magnificent Aluvise to whom Cornaro writes in January 1551, but here we enter into pure speculation.

113 [Cornaro:] "Now I will come to the bequests. And if I do not have for you, my dear friends and servants, such a large show [of money] that I have made in other wills, it is not then because I do not love you in the way I have always loved you, but I am compelled not to do so given the large number of my grandchildren, whose number is now at eleven with the one being born in a month; and I am certain that in 5 or 6 years, by the Grace of God, it will be 15, for which I am naturally compelled to be austere with you" (Sambin, "I testamenti …," [in *Italia Medioevale* …, IX (1966)], p. 376).

between that house and the Odeo.[114] Curiously enough, he does not alter his will either after the death of his son-in-law or after those of his two grandsons, but waits until his final days to draw up another one. Here, contrary to what he had said in the preceding ones, he designates that he be buried at Santo and not at the Church of San Bartolamio in Venice; in addition, he leaves to Giacomo Alvise, as the only bequest, the house in Padua because, being the grandson already "wealthy by reason of marriage," he can readily maintain the many expenses associated with it.

In his last will, he also provides the arrangements for his own funeral:

> I wish my burial to be in this church of the Santo, in the place I designated and decided it should be. And for the day of my burial I do not want there to be great amounts spent on appearances and things, but humble, and that the number of Masses given be decided by my commissioners and so too in what is given in charity to the poor of the area. And I also wish them to decide on the Masses spoken at the church of Codevigo and the charity given to the poor of that villa.[115]

There is no mention of what he had stated in the *Eulogy*:

> And to remain helpful even after his death, he pledged that [his body] be opened to make known how well a sober life had conserved him on the inside overall. He wanted his body to be buried together with the bones of several of his friends, and he did not want a showy funeral. (139)

---

114 [Cornaro:] "And because I do not doubt that one day there will be a fire in that part of the stables, which could easily happen and cause much damage, my idea therefore is for that part to be torn down and redone – since it is my design – so that the stable will not be under the rooms but in the courtyard where the hens are held, and kept away with respect to a fire. And besides, I want it done this way because the loggia will be done in the courtyard, similar to the one in the rooms of the octagonal and the other 2 turned to face the old house. And so the courtyard will become a square and will be very beautiful [...] As for the rest of the building that goes toward the path, as can be seen in the model, I do not want anyone to feel obliged to do it because it will be rather expensive; although I hope that Giacomo Alvise will [do it], because then he will have the most beautiful house of any city in Italy," (Sambin, "I testamenti ...," [in *Italia Medioevale ...*, IX (1966)], p. 379). This last project of Cornaro's was never realized, instead, with the passing of the centuries, the house underwent such extensive restructuring as to render its original state unrecognizable.

115 P. Sambin, "I testamenti ...," [in *Italia Medioevale ...*, IX (1966)], p. 382.

This sounds like one of the countless number of "likely stories" by Cornaro, but it is true that he could not have let anything so patently false be said at his own funeral. In any event, everyone knew about his wish to be reunited for all eternity with his friends, as Vasari attests:

> Messer Luigi had designated that in his own tomb, which would be made, he be put to rest together with Giovanni Maria [Falconetto] and the *facetissimo* poet Ruzzante with whom he was the closest, and who lived and died in his house: but I do not know if what Cornaro had designated was then carried out.[116]

Not even we know, because the tombs of these three most extraordinary Renaissance men of Padua have never again been found. And who knows if this might not just be Cornaro's ultimate inspired joke?

Padua,
September 1981

---

116 *"Vite de' più eccellenti Pittori Scultori e Architetti scritte da Giorgio Vasari pittore e architetto aretino* (Venice 1828), t. IX, pp. 225–6.

Writings on the Sober Life

The Art and Grace of Living Long*

ALVISE CORNARO

E chi è quello che potesse haver a noia un tanto bene,
tanto contento et tanta gratia, come haverò io?
La qual cosa avvenirebbe ad ogni altro homo che tenesse
la vita che ho tenuta io, la qual si può tenere da ogn'uno …

Amorevole essortazione

And who could be troubled by so great a good, so
great a happiness and so great a grace as will be mine?
It is something every other man would have who
follows the life I have led, which anyone can follow …

Loving Exhortation

---

* Notes on pages 72–182 are by this translator.

Letter to Bishop Cornelio Musso
by Bernardino Tomitano

To the Most Reverend and Most Worthy Monsignor Cornelio Bishop of Bitonto[1]

The reverence and love, the former as great as the latter is glorious, which the Magnificent Messer Luigi[*] Cornaro conveys to your Most Reverend Lordship, has brought me to the task I presently undertake, to make known under your honoured name[**] this brief work no less beautiful than it is enjoyable, no less enjoyable than it is beneficial to the world. On the one hand I knew about this honest desire on the part of the Author, and on the other he showed his no less infinite diffidence. Therefore, eager with this humble gesture of gratitude to fulfill his desire and to direct part of his labour to where neither more highly nor more honourably it could be placed, I pray you accept this very precious gift that he and I together respectfully offer to you. To you, in truth, this offering was due, to you alone this sacrifice of a sober and moderate life pertains, your Lordship being – in addition to your infinite other virtues, in part natural and in part elected [by your will] – enhanced by this most beautiful part of living in a sober manner and in moderation. This is shown by the divine operations of your

---

1 Cornelio Musso (1511–1574), Cornaro's much beloved and close friend – like a "son" – author of religious texts, was "the most famous among preachers of the 16th century," an extraordinary orator, called the "Italian Demosthenes." He delivered the inaugural oration at the Council of Trent (1545). Also see Milani's lengthy note on Musso in *Scritti sulla vita sobria: Elogio e Lettere*, "Prima edizione critica a cura di Marisa Milani" (Venice: Corbo e Fiore Editori, 1983), pp. 75–6n1 (the Milani edition is cited herein as *Scritti …*, this Da Ponte edition is cited herein as *Sober …*,).

* Luigi = Alvise = Aluvise. The spelling is a variation on the Latin Clovis. Also see "Terminology," *s.v.*

** *under your honoured name*: in dedication to you.

undaunted spirit [*animo valoroso*],[2] which – not aggravated by a heavy body or tyrannized by temptations of hunger, or, finally, not oppressed by an excessive desire for food – every day imparts more clear examples of pilgrim works, which, as once they were utilized for the good of the most brilliant studies of Italy, are now thus expended for the benefit of and in tribute to the Holy Church. It does me good to witness that your Lordship has for no other reason, after Divine assistance, maintained the health of your body quite successfully in my judgment (if we look at the long fasts and fatigue that your smaller frame has withstood), the result of always having been prudent and disciplined; it is, therefore, of no little authority or confirmation to give to this work the testimony of your life and of your strengths that so valiantly defended against contrary accidents.[3] Nevertheless, let every man know who will read of these things that I do not publish this volume as a physician nor as a medical book, given that the Author has never practised this art as a profession.[4] Nor was it his intention to enrich the greatly vast Ocean of Medicine with this small current of his branch, as it was something he knew very well had not been overlooked by more than one classical writer, that is, in elaborating and in broadening the terms of this art. It was truly my sole intention to make known in this way the value and virtue of the gentleman, born in a free city, his steadfastness in defending himself from the siren of the senses, his patience in abstaining from foods delectable to the taste, his fortitude in not overeating what is good, and finally, the victory achieved by that very sobriety against those delights, which enticed and lured him to serve and obey them. Through all of this it will be known how powerful Nature is in revealing her secrets to another without the aid of art [medical profession] and finally, how many would benefit a great deal from the knowledge and

---

2 *undaunted spirit* (*animo valoroso*): e.g., intrepid spirit/soul, valiant heart, daring spirit. Spirit, here, is the sense of "to give life to something." On *animo*, see "Note on the Translation," or see "Terminology," *s.v.*

3 *Accident* (versus essence): that which is non-essential to the substance of a thing is an accident. It is an attribute or property which does not affect the substance of the thing. For example, no matter the colour of a person's skin (accident), he or she remains a human being (essence).

4 *art*: here refers to a discipline; for example, its particular theories and practices, as in the liberal arts, political arts, military arts etc., which is practical and variable, versus "science" and its (in theory) invariable and universal principles. Tomitano speaks of the medical arts.

experience of one man. But not to be more tiresome to your most Reverend Lordship, I pray on this humble occasion you vouch for yourself how much the spirit undaunted of Messer Luigi broadens [the medical arts], and how much my own modest strengths can do, we being, in our will as in our judgment, compliant in our love and observance of you, and pray for your happiness.

Padua, 10th day of November, in the year M.D.LVIII [1558].
Most Devoted Servant to Your Most Reverend Lordship,
Bernardin Tomitano[5]

---

5 Bernardino Tomitano (1517–1576) was a physician, scholar, philosopher, and founder of the Accademia letteraria, familiar with the works of Ficino, Galen, and Michele Savonarola, his own writings include a work on pestilence, "*Consiglio sopra la peste di Veneti.*" A close friend of Cornaro, he at times acted as his editor. For more on Tomitano, see Milani's lengthy note in *Scritti* ..., pp. 76–7n1.

A Treatise on the Sober Life by the Magnificent Messer Luigi Cornaro,[6] Noble Venetian

To be sure, over time a man's habit becomes his nature,[7] obliging him to use it either well or poorly. Similarly, we see that in many things habit is stronger than reason, which we cannot deny; rather, we often see that a good person using and practising a habit with someone wicked, becomes wicked. The good person he once was becomes bad. We also see the opposite, that is, since a good habit can easily change to bad, so it is that the bad can return to good; because then we find that this wicked person – who once was good – practising [a habit] with a good person will himself return to being good. But it cannot come about if not for the power of habit, which is truly great. And that habit would have so great an influence in Italy is, according to my observations and thoughts, owing to three bad practices introduced not long ago, rather, within my lifetime: the first is flattery and its rituals, the second is living according to Lutheran beliefs[8] – to which, some, in great error, are becoming

---

6 On the "fate" of Alvise Cornaro's *Vita sobria* in English, see the essay "Immortality ...," included here by Milani. For biographical information on Cornaro, see "Intro.," or see "Foreword"; in Italian, also see "Corner, Alvise" in *Dizionario Biografico degli Italiani* (1983), Vol. XXIX; or see, for example, *Alvise Cornaro e il suo tempo*, the catalogue for the exhibit, ed. Lionello Puppi (Padua: Comune di Padova, 1980).

7 This has also been interpreted as "second nature," which is not stated in the Italian.

8 Martin Luther (1483–1546), German, was a preacher and Bible scholar, declared a heretic in 1521 after his "Ninety-Five Theses" (1917) attacked Roman Catholic "abuses." Contributing to this crisis were reformers such as John Calvin (Jean Cauvin), (1509–1564), and, according to Peter Harrison, "the Reformed Church, the Radical Reformation, and, not least, the reforms that took place with the Catholic Church itself" for whom "[t]he crisis of religion, in other words, was to a considerable degree a crisis of authority." "Philosophy and the Crisis of Religion," in *The Cambridge Companion to Renaissance Philosophy*, ed. James Hankins (Cambridge, UK: University of Cambridge Press, 2007), p. 235.

habituated – and the third is crapula.[9] These three vices, or rather cruel monsters of human life, have reduced our times to deterring the integrity of civil life, the religion of the soul, and the health of the body. I resolved to address this last one and to demonstrate that it is abuse, and so be rid of it if possible, because in regard to Lutheran beliefs and the [other], which is flattery, I am certain that soon enough some noble spirit will take up the burden of censuring and removing them from the world. And so I hope that before I die, I see these three abuses eliminated and made extinct in Italy, and I see her restored to her beautiful and blessed customs.

Returning to the subject I intended to discuss, crapula, I say it is a bad thing that has smothered the sober life and very much stifled it; and though everyone knows that crapula comes from the vice of overindulgence and a sober life from the virtue of Continence,[10] nevertheless, crapula is looked upon as something virtuous and honourable, and a sober life as dishonourable and for parsimonious men. And it all comes from the power of habit, introduced by the senses and appetites, which have greatly tempted and inebriated men, who, having strayed from the good path, have taken to following the worst one. This leads [men], without their being aware, to unknown and deadly ailments that age them,

---

9 Cornaro uses the word "crapula," which is an excess in drinking or eating. The Latin *crapula* arrives from 'the Greek *kraipalē*) or *kraipälh*, "drunken headache or nausea, the result of a drunken debauch," and "the sickness or indisposition following a drunken or gluttonous debauch," *Oxford Enlish Dictionary* CD 2nd ed. [herein, *OED*]. "[D]runkenness caused men to be 'insane,' and too much food in the stomach turned 'the power of nature' away from the head," N. Arikha, *Passions and Tempers: A History of the Humours* (New York: HarperCollins, 2007) [herein, *Passions …*,], p. 125. "Crapula," as used here, is strictly in regard to a person who consumes a "superfluous" amount of food or drink, with the consequence of an ill effect. "There are four powers, which every creature and plant shares: absorption, retention, transformation and rejection of whatever is superfluous. Superfluity can be divided into two types: either superfluous in quantity or quality." Mark Grant, *Galen on Food and Diet* (London: Routledge, 2000), p. 55. Also see writings on the ancient medical theorist and natural philosopher Alcmaeon of Croton (fifth? century BCE) on food excess, and the imbalances of bodily elements (*isonomia*) that lead to illness. Fragments from his work [on nature, 450? BCE] and theories on the immortality of the soul, physiology, and dietary norms, were known to Plato, Aristotle, Hippocrates, and Galen, among others.
10 *Continence* signifies a holding back, said of passions, desires, etc., self-restraint versus *incontinence*, which here means a lack of restraint, given to abandon, especially of the sexual appetite. Also see "Terminology,": *Continence*, and *Virtue* (*virtù*), on its sense of "manly" qualities.

and before reaching the age of forty they have become decrepit. This is contrary to what a sober life did, which kept them prosperous well into their eighties, before it was forced out by this deadly crapula.[11]

O wretched and unhappy Italy, do you not see how many of your people this crapula kills each year? There have been so many, yet fewer have died of pestilence when at its worst,[12] or of the sword or gunfire throughout her many armed conflicts. This is because Italy's true armed conflicts are her immoral banquets, now common practice, which are so immense and so unsustainable that tables cannot hold the infinite number of foods placed on them and so the dishes must be piled one on top of the other.[13] Who could ever live in such chaos and disorder? Do something, for the love of God, as I am sure there is no vice more displeasing to His Almighty than this. Drive out this new death, rather this heretofore unnamed pestilence, in the same way scourge was driven out in times past, which once doing great harm now does very little, in fact, almost none, owing to the good practice introduced by good prevention. There is still a remedy for being rid of this crapula, a remedy that can be used by everyone on their own, as men living in harmony with the

---

11 *Prosperous:* to prosper or to flourish, to be successful and happy in life (*eudaemonia*). Its variant, *prosperity* is used both in a material sense and to signify the physical well-being and "happiness" of man.

12 A possible reference to the Bubonic Plague of 1347/1348, lasting some four years, estimated to have killed a third of the population of Europe. Regular outbreaks continued, for example, in Germany in 1566 (the year Cornaro died); Italy, including Venice, in 1575/1576; London, England in 1665, and Marseille, France in 1720. Preventative measures, reputed to have originated in Italy during the 1350s, were enacted to restrict travel into and out of Italy, isolate the healthy, and segregate the infected in *lazzaretti*, places of quarantine originally for maritime travelers (some were specifically used or built for those with leprosy).

13 "One banquet laid out for fifty-four people, during Lent so there was no meat, consisted of over a dozen courses including anywhere from fifteen to fifty-four individual servings of 140 separate foods. This comes to over 2,500 plates," Ken Albala, *Eating Right in the Renaissance* (Berkeley: University of California Press, 2002), p. 213. That observation is found in *Banchetti, compositioni di vivande, et apparecchio generale* (Ferrara: De Buglhat e Hucher, 1549), written by the remarkable Cristoforo da Messisbugo (late 1400s?–1548), who later became Count Palatine and whose "obsessive eye" details his life of some thirty years overseeing the Este Court in Ferrara as its *maggiordomo* or court administrator. His many duties included those of overseeing the menu, diplomacy, finance, and as "theatrical impresario." Luciano Chiappini, *La Corte estense alla metà del Cinquecento* (c1984), or see Ken Albala, *The Banquet: Dining in the Great Courts of Late Renaissance Europe* (Urbana: University of Illinois Press, 2007).

simplicity of Nature, which teaches us to be content with little, by following the way of blessed Continence and that of Divine Reason, and by becoming accustomed to eating only what is needed to sustain life knowing that more [eating] means complete infirmity and death, and that it is simply out of pleasure for the taste,[14] which lasts but a moment, yet in the long run causes displeasure and damage to the body, and in the end kills the body along with the soul. I have seen many friends die of this [form of] pestilence at an early age, bright of mind and kind of nature, who, if alive, would have graced the world and much to my happiness I would be enjoying their company, for I am now left in such sorrow without them.

Therefore, to avert further damage to come, with this brief discourse I have resolved to make known how crapula is abuse and that we can easily be rid of it and introduce the sober life in its place, to where it once was. And I wish to do this even more willingly, since many bright-minded young people, knowing that crapula is vice, have urged me to do so, because they have seen their fathers die at an early age and yet they see me so healthy and prosperous at the old age of eighty-one years.[15] And because it is an age they still hope to reach, and because Nature does not prohibit us from living for a very long time, and because it is in fact at that age when it is possible to exercise prudence and with little notable difference enjoy the fruits of other virtues – because then the senses are discarded and in their place man gives himself wholly over to reason – they have implored me to be so kind and tell them the method I have followed to reach this age. Seeing them filled with such honest desire, and in order to help them, together with others who wish to read my discourse, I will write on it, stating the reasons that forced me to abandon crapula and to embrace a sober life, recounting the entire method I followed in doing so, and relating how that good habit then operated in me. It will thus be clearly understood how easy it is to be rid of the abuse

---

14 Taste, the sense that permits us to perceive and distinguish flavours, also the pleasure and delight, or satisfaction, of the palate, of the spirit or senses. See *OED*, *s.v.* Taste also relates to the *complexion* (or constitution) of a person, in as much as it can change that complexion. See below, note 20; also see "Terminology," *s.v.*

15 In 1558, Cornaro is either seventy-four or seventy-six years of age (see below, note 51). In regard to the discrepancies in Cornaro's age and the absence of anyone to contradict him, Milani speculates that it may be owing to a strategy of good marketing, because both family and others wished to maintain and promote the image of Cornaro as the very aged living exemplar of sobriety and longevity, see *Scritti* ..., p. 98n21; also see herein the essay "Immortality ... ."

of crapula; and in conclusion, I will include the many uses and benefits to be had from a sober life.

For that reason I say that, unfortunately, infirmity not only had a very forceful beginning in me but it also made not a little progress, which is the reason I abandoned crapula, at which I was very adept. So that because of [crapula] and my poor complexion[16] – since my stomach is very cool and very moist[17] – I came down with all sorts of ailments, that is, pain in the stomach and often in my side,[18] the beginning of gout and much worse, along with a low fever that was almost continuous, but above all an unsettled stomach and a perpetual thirst. For this poor or rather terrible disposition, there was nothing for me to hope for except to die from the torments and afflictions of my life; my being as far from the end owing to Nature, as being near to it owing to the disordered terms of my life. Thus finding myself in such poor condition, between the ages of thirty-five and forty years, and having tried everything to regain my health with nothing that helped, the doctors informed me that for my ills there was but one medicine, available whenever I would resolve to use it and to continue unwaveringly with its use. It was the life of sobriety and order. And, they added, it held the greatest virtue and strength, as much virtue and strength as the other – being in every way contrary to it – by which I mean crapula and a disordered life, whose powers I understood very well, since it was by their disorders I had become completely infirm.

---

16 Complexion, arriving from classical and later Galenic "complexion theory" of the humours, is the state of a living body, "the costitutive essence of it." The term, as used here, involves the proportional balance (cf., *isonomia*, or *eukrasia*) in the body of the properties of cold or hot, moist or dry, combined with the four elements, four humours, and (with Galen) the four temperaments. Its predisposition to disease results from a disproportion or imbalance of humours (*dyskrasia*). *UTET, s.v.* See, for example, N. Arikha, *Passions ...,* . Cf., for example, "temperament" in Nancy Siraisi, *The Clock and the Mirror ...: Girolamo Cardano and Renaissance Medicine* (Princeton, NJ: Princeton University Press, 1997), or "complexion" in Nancy Siraisi, *Medieval and Early Renaissance Medicine: An introduction to Knowledge and Practice* (Chicago: University of Chicago Press, 1990). Also see "Terminology," *s.v.*

17 *Radical moisture.* Considered the "life oil" or essence of a person, in combination with the heat of the body it is continuously consumed throughout life, lasting, ideally, well into old age before finally being depleted (out of resolution) at a natural death. Semen, classically thought to be produced from blood, and later for the physician and philosopher Avicenna (Persia, 980–1037), it became the fourth moisture, or radical moisture. Also see "Terminology": *Coitus, Semen.*

18 Possible reference to an ulcer, or a hernia on one or both sides.

But I had not yet been reduced to such a condition that an ordered life, operating contrary to a disordered one, could not completely free me of [disorders], and that this was still possible. Because we see that such a life, and order, does in fact keep men of poor complexion and decrepit age in good health, as long as they follow it; since its contrary has the power to make ill someone who has a perfect complexion – [while] at his youngest and most vigorous age – and keep him in that state for the longest period of time. And it is for a natural reason, which requires that from contrary forms of living, contrary operations be produced; with [an ordered life] mimicking in this, still as art, Nature's proficiency of being able – together by means of this art – to correct the faults and defects of Nature; something that can clearly be seen in agriculture and other similar things. Furthermore, they said that if I did not make use of that medicine right away, within a few months it could no longer be of help to me and within a few months after that I would die. Myself, rather displeased at dying at such a youthful age and finding myself continually tormented by illness, and having heard these beautiful and natural reasons, I was persuaded that from order and disorder the said contrary effects would necessarily come to be, and reanimated by hope I resolved not to die but to emerge from my torments and to give myself over to living a regulated life. At that point, they informed me of the way I should conduct myself, with it being understood that I would have nothing to eat or drink except for the food or wine for the so-called infirm, and in the case of one or the other, in small quantity. In truth, they had already asked this of me before, but at that time, wanting to live by my own rules and finding myself, let us say, satisfied by those foods, I could not help but satisfy myself and I ate the things that pleased me. Similarly, feeling a burning thirst because of the pain, I could not help but drink the wine I liked, and in great quantity, without mentioning it at all to the doctors, just as all infirm people do. But since I had resolved to be *continente* [restrained] and reasonable, seeing that it was not a difficult thing – rather, it was a duty proper to man – I took up that way of living, and I was never afterward disordered in anything. In doing so, and within a few days, I noticed that such a life was greatly beneficial to me, and by following it, within less than a year (though it may seem incredible to some) I had recovered from every one of my infirmities.

Restored thus to health, I took to considering the virtue of order, telling myself that if order had the force to overcome the many things that were bad in me, it would then have greater force to conserve me while in good health, and to help my poor complexion and to comfort my very weak stomach. I therefore diligently undertook to learn which foods would serve my purpose, and I first resolved to experience whether or not the ones that tasted good would benefit or harm me, to discover if that proverb, which I already thought to be true and is universally accepted as being very true – rather, it is the foundation of all the *sensuali* who follow their appetites[19] – was in fact true: which says, that which tastes good, nourishes and benefits.[20] In doing so I found it to be false, because to me a very sharp cold wine tasted good, so too melons and other fruits, raw salads, fish, pork, *tortas* [cakes or pies: sweet, or savoury], legume soups, pasta, and other similar foods that delighted me enormously and yet all were harmful to me. Thus, having found the proverb to be false, it was then false. And so based upon my experience, I stayed away from those types of food and wine, or from drinking it cold, and I selected wine suitable to my stomach; drinking it in the amount I knew I could easily digest. I did the same with food, in quality[21] as in quantity, becoming accustomed to my appetite never being satisfied by either food or drink, so that I would rise from the table while still hungry and still thirsty, in keeping with the saying: not being sated with food is a study in health.[22] And

---

19 *sensuali … appetites*: *sensual* used as a substantive here (also in English, signifying beings that seek only to satisfy sense driven needs. The *OED* defines sensuals as "beings capable only of sensation, brutes … The souls of men and angels are reasonable; … and the sensuals (as beasts and such like) not so." Also see *Dizionario della lingua italiana* (Battaglia, UTET), *s.v.* Here, Cornaro likens the *sensuali* to animals who satisfy, in excess, their appetites for food, drink, and sex. Also see "Terminology": *Sensual.*

    Appetite, as used here refers to the desire, craving, inclination or disposition toward attaining something, thus a personal preference or likeness. In Scholasticism, it applies to all strivings.

20 Proverb: "*quello che sa buono nutrisce et giova.*" With regard to this maxim: "Foods we like, those similar to us (that is, more like human flesh) and apt for retention, are embraced or hugged by the stomach. This idea informed the Arabist position that what tastes good is necessarily more nourishing because it is better processed. The agglutinative property of some foods, like bread, was also thought to keep everything in place." K. Albala, *Eating Right*, p. 59. Also see N. Siraisi, *Medieval … .*

21 *Quality*: here, signifies an "attribute, property, special feature or characteristic [that is] … primary, secondary, etc.," *OED.*

22 Proverb: "il non satiarsi di cibi è uno studio di sanità." Milani refers the reader to Lucio Fauno's Italian translation (from Latin) of Marsilio Ficino (1433–1499): "egli (possendosi comodamente fare) per mangiare si vuole aspettare di avere fame, e non si vuol bere, fin che non ci chiami la sete, et si dee alzare l'huomo da tavola con qualche desiderio di amendue queste cose, e si vuol fuggire, come il serpe, la troppa satietà di loro, e quel'affanno, e fastidio, che suole sentire chi ha troppo pieno el ventre," Fauno, *Marsilio Ficino. De le tre vite …*, (1479) 15*vr* [cited herein as *Tre vite…*: [Before eating (being convenient to do so) one waits for hunger to come, and does not drink until thirst calls, and man should rise from the table with some desire left for both these things and avoid,

for these reasons, ridding myself in this way of crapula and disorders, I dedicated myself to a sober and regulated life, which primarily operated in me in the way I mentioned before, that is, within less than a year I was free of every illness that once had a strong beginning in me, rather, that had progressed so far as to be almost incurable. A further benefit was that I no longer became ill, as had always happened before when a year could never pass while following that other way of living – the one of the senses – without my falling ill with a very strange fever, which had often brought me to death's door.

Freed of this once again, I then became very healthy and have remained so from that time until now, for no other reason than the fact that I have never lacked order, which has operated its infinite virtue; thus, the food I always ate and the wine I drank – being those suitable to my complexion and of suitable quantity – in the same way they had left their virtue in my body, so too they left [my body] without difficulty, not having first generated within me any bad humour.[23] And by always following that path, I have always been, and I find myself now as was already said (God granting), very healthy. It is true that other than the two orders mentioned above, which I have always followed in eating and drinking, and which are very important – that is, to eat only the amount my stomach can easily digest and nothing that I know is unsuitable – I have also guarded against suffering the cold and heat, overextending myself, interrupting my usual sleep, excessive coitus,[24] remaining where

---

like [avoiding] a serpent, overindulging in them, and the worry and trouble, which happens only to someone whose belly is too full]," see *Scritti ...*, p. 83n5. And cf. *Three Books on Life*. Trans. and notes Carol V. Kaske and John R. Clark (Binghampton, NY: Medieval & Renaissance Texts and Studies in conjunction with the Renaissance Society of America, 1989), p. 137 [cited herein as *Three Books ...,*].

23 Certain combinations of foods with certain humours in the body can produce adverse or bad humours. "Both good and bad varieties of each can be produced from various foods and internal processes. For example, pork might be converted into good humors in a body strong enough to digest it but in a weaker system might generate only 'raw' humors," K. Albala, *Eating Right ...*, p. 49.

24 "Coitus," Ficino writes, "is damaging to the stomach; especially if done while full, or when very hungry," (*Tre vite ...*, 16v). "This same coitus is worse in the day, and surer at night, if the one in the day is not however followed right away with food, and if after the one at night there is no need to exercise and stay awake" from Cornelio Celso (in the Appendix to Galeno, *Delli Mezzi ...*, 157v), excerpted from a note in *Scritti ...*, pp. 84–5n6.

   Avicenna writes: "If any sperm should flow away through sexual intercourse beyond that which nature tolerates, it is more harmful than if forty times as much blood should pour forth," (N. Arikha, *Passions ...*, p. 124). Also see "Terminology." *s.v.*

the air is bad, and suffering either the wind or sun, which – also these – are powerful disorders. And as it happens, it is not difficult to guard against them, the desire of a reasonable man tending more towards life and health than the gratification of doing what will ultimately harm him.

As much as I was able, I also guarded against those things from which we cannot easily defend ourselves: these are melancholy, hate, and other perturbations of the soul [*animo*],[25] which seem to have the greatest power over our bodies. And yet I have not been able to guard as well against either one or another of these sorts of disorders, many of which I have incurred at different times, not to mention all of them at present. But this [event] has helped me in this way, in that, owing to my experience I have understood that they do not really hold a great deal of power, nor can they do a great deal of harm to bodies regulated by the two orders of the mouth discussed above. I can therefore say in truth that whoever observes these two principal ones will suffer little from other disorders. But, prior to me, this belief was proven by Galen,[26] a truly great physician, who affirms that all other disorders did little harm to him because he guarded against them by means of the two [orders] of the mouth; hence, he never became ill due to other ailments if not for only a day. And it truly is as he says, for which I offer myself as living proof, since many more who know me and know how frequently I have suffered the cold, heat, and other similar disorders at other times, have likewise seen me – owing to the various accidents that have befallen me – with my spirit [*animo*] tested. Nevertheless, they know that these

---

25 On *animo*, see "Note on Translation"; also see "Terminology": *Animo* and *Perturbation*.

26 Claudius Galenus (129/30?–199/216? CE), or Galen of Pergamon, was a physician-surgeon, anatomist, philosopher, philologist, and scholar, who later resided in Rome while serving emperors Marcus Aurelius, Commodus, then Severus; his work elaborates Hippocratic (460 BCE) concepts, and he is renowned for his findings on health and disease (pathology). Galen was known for his use of medical observation and experimental research; his findings on animal dissection, blood, and nerves, in addition to his scholarship, remained pre-eminent, influencing medical thought for centuries. A prodigious author (in Greek), not all of his works have survived. Certain texts were first translated from the original Greek into Syriac (then Arabic) principally by two Syriac scholars, Sergius of Res 'Ayna (d. 536?) and the physician and scientist, Hunayn Ibn Ishaq (809–873), known in the Latin West as Joannitius – as well as into other languages, including English. The translation from extant Greek texts into Latin (1821–1833) by Carolus G. Kühn (1754–1840) consists of some 20 volumes. Other works of Galen are found in the ongoing academic project *Corpus Medicorum Graecorum* on ancient medical texts. Cornaro would have had access to a 1549 Italian translation, see "Introduction," p. 10n17.

[accidents] did little harm to me, just as they know that many others, who did not lead a sober and regulated life, were harmed a great deal by them; one of whom was my own brother, and other members of my household, who, trusting in their good complexions, did not maintain a regulated life. And this caused them the most grievous harm, because in them the accidents of the spirit had the greatest power,[27] and the pain and melancholy they suffered was too great after having seen several lawsuits brought against me, for considerable sums of money, by powerful and important men. And doubting that I could win against them, they were overcome with melancholy humour, which is always plentiful in those bodies of an unregulated life, and this one [his brother's melancholy] altered in manner and increased so much that it made him die before his time.[28] But I did not suffer any ill effect, because in me there was no surfeit of that humour, rather, taking heart myself, it made me believe that God – in order to make known how steadfast and undaunted I was – had caused these lawsuits to be brought against me and that I would win them to my benefit and honour, as was the case. Because in the end [the experience] brought victory along with much glory and advantage, for which in my heart I felt the greatest consolation while at the same time it did not have any power to harm me. Therefore, we see that neither melancholy nor other affect can harm the body of one who leads a sober and ordered life.

But I will add that these same maladies do not have any power over [regulated] bodies, save for a little ill effect, nor do they cause anything more than a little pain. And I know this to be true, because at the age of seventy I had such an experience – which usually happens when travelling at great speed in a carriage – for, by chance, the carriage tipped over and was dragged along its side a fair distance before the horses could stop. Still being inside, I was left with pain everywhere, around my head and all my body from the injuries and thumps received; what is more, my leg and arm were injured. Brought back to my home, my family immediately sent for the doctors, and once they had arrived – seeing

---

27　According to Hippocratic thought, and Aristotle, *pneuma* – Greek for air, wind or breath (with the Stoics it becomes spirit) – is essential for maintaining the vitality of the body as a whole. Any bad pneuma-spirit entering the body affects the various centres of spirit (natural, vital, animal), causing disorders. *Accidents* or attributes of the soul, or spirit, include acts such as reasoning, striving, or worrying.

28　Cornaro's brother Giacomo died in 1541, his close friend Beolco (Ruzzante) in 1542 at about forty years old.

me so battered and in such poor condition and in consideration of my age – they concluded that although by this misfortune I would die within three days, they could provide me with two treatments. One was to draw my blood, and the other was to purge me and obviate the possibility of altering my humours, which they thought could become very active at any time and cause a terrible fever. I, however, knew that my regulated life, which I had already been maintaining for many years, had so conquered, tamed, and checked my humours that they could not be much activated by this. I did not want to be bled nor to take other medicines, but only to have my leg and arm put right, and have some of their oils rubbed on me, which they said would do me good. And so it was, without the need of any other treatment – as I knew – that I recovered from this [event] without any other problem or alteration, something seemingly miraculous to the doctors. One must therefore conclude, whoever follows a sober and regulated life, and not a disordered one, will suffer little harm from other disorders or unfortunate accidents. Yet I firmly conclude – largely owing to the experience I have recently undergone – that those [disorders] of living are fatal disorders. I then confirmed it four years ago when I was induced, on the advice of my doctors and the prompting of friends and the concern of my own family, to endure one [disorder] – which in truth was much more significant, as was later seen, than first thought – which was to increase the quantity of food I ordinarily ate, and which reduced me to a deadly illness. But it is something that, since it is fitting to mention here and may benefit another, I am happy to recount.

So it was that my dearest relatives and friends, who love and care for me a great deal – and moved by their beautiful and kind love, and seeing that I ate very little – together with the doctors told me that the food I was taking was insufficient to sustain an old and declining age such as mine, which, at that point, not only had to be conserved but had to increase in strength and vigour. And being something that can only be done with food, it was thus absolutely necessary that I eat much more. I, on the other hand, set out my reasoning for them, which is that Nature is content with little, and that with this little I had conserved myself for many years and that this habit had changed my nature; and that it was more logical – with the passing of the years and with my diminishing prosperity – that I be decreasing and not increasing the amount of food, since the strength of my stomach is naturally becoming less effective by the hour, for which I saw no reason to agree to such an increase. To support my reasoning, I offered these two natural and absolutely true proverbs: the one that says, whoever wishes to eat a lot need eat a little, which is said only because eating little leads to a long life and living long leads to eating a lot; and the other, that the food left uneaten is more beneficial, because after eating, what has already been eaten is of no benefit. And yet, neither of these proverbs nor any reason I gave to them were of any help to me, because with every passing hour they besieged me more intently, and so as not to appear obstinate or more of a physician than the physicians and above all to please my family, who very much wished this for me since they believed such an increase conserves *virtù*,[29] I agreed to increase my food – but only by two ounces more. And while before – with the bread, egg yolk, meat, and soup – I ate what in all weighed twelve short ounces,[30] I then increased it to fourteen, and whereas before I drank fourteen ounces of wine, I increased these to sixteen. Within ten days, this increase and this disorder began to affect me and the happy person I once was became melancholic and choleric to the point where everything bothered me, and being always in a strange mood, I did not know what to do or say. By the twelfth day, I was struck with tremendous pain in my side that lasted twenty-two hours, in addition to which I had a terrible fever that lasted thirty-five days and as many nights without ever going away; though in truth after fifteen days it was lower. But at the time with all of this, I could not sleep for fifteen minutes, and everyone thought I would die. Yet I freed myself (by God's Grace) through my order alone, even though I was seventy-eight years old and it was the coldest season of the year, which was extremely cold, and with my body as emaciated as it could be. And I am entirely convinced I escaped death only because of the great order I had maintained for so many years, during which time I never had any illness except for being a little indisposed for one or two days. It is because the order of many years, to which I refer, had prevented any dominant or malignant humours from generating within me, and without them being generated, for me to age then in that wretchedness and malignity that happens to those bodies living without order. Therefore, not finding among my humours any old malignancies, which are what kill men, but only the one newly introduced by that new disorder, my illness, though most serious, did not have the force to kill me.

––––––––––––––––––––

29 *Virtù* here refers to strength, power, and manly traits. Also see "Terminology," *s.v.* on its variations.

30 A *sottile* ounce or *short* ounce equals twenty-five grams; a *grossa* ounce or *full* ounce equals forty-three grams. See "Intro.," p. 22n38, and see "Immortality …," p. 201n31.

I was alive for this reason and no other, and so it can be seen how great is the power and virtue of order, and how great the [power] of disorder that within a few days had caused such a terrible illness in me, given that a sober and ordered life had kept me healthy for so many years. It seemed to me all the more reason that if the world conserves itself with order and our life is nothing but the harmony and order of the four elements in the body,[31] then it is order itself that should conserve and maintain our life; and conversely, it means that life is broken down by illness operating to the contrary, or is corrupted by death. Order more readily teaches discipline. Order renders the army victorious and, finally, order maintains the City, the Family and the Kingdom itself. Thus, I resolve that an ordered life is none other than the most assured reason and foundation for a healthy and long life; therefore, it must be said that it is the one and only true medicine, and whoever considers this at length should conclude the same thing. Thus, when the physician visits one who is ill, he reminds him that this is the first medicine and commits him to living a life of order. And the patient, released from his care, and since he has regained his health – and wanting to remain so – commits to keeping an ordered life. There is no doubt that if he were to maintain that life he could never be ill again, because it removes all the causes for illness, thus he would no longer have need of either doctors or medicine; rather, by putting his mind [*mente*] to what he must do, he would be his own physician and the most perfect one; as, in truth, man cannot be a perfect physician for anyone but himself. And the reason is because each person can learn through his various experiences about his own complexion perfectly well, along with its most occult [hidden] properties, and which wine and which food suits his stomach. These are things we can never really know about another, things that only through our own hard work we can know about ourselves, since it takes a long time to acquire and learn from these different experiences. And these experiences are more than necessary, because man is more diverse in his

---

31 The classical relation between the humours and the elements (Empedocles) in a medical application is attributed to Hippocrates (c.460–c.370 BCE), continuing with Galen and his addition of complexions or temperaments. The four classical elements and their corresponding humours and complexions are earth (black bile, melancholic), air (blood, sanguine), fire (yellow bile, choleric), and water (phlegm, phlegmatic). A fifth element, Aether, was also considered (Plato, Aristotle) as the quintessence of celestial bodies (stars = planets) and the cosmos. See for example, N. Siraisi, *Medieval ...*, or see N. Arikha, *Passions ... .*

nature and his stomach than he is in his appearance. Who would believe an old wine, older than a year, would be harmful to my stomach and that a new one would be beneficial; and that pepper, reputed to be a hot spice, would not have that hot effect in me, since I feel more warmed and comforted by cinnamon? Which doctor could have told me about these two occult properties of mine, when I myself, only after lengthy observation, have become aware of them? And so it is, no one can be a perfect physician to someone else.

Accordingly, not having a better physician than himself or a better medicine than an ordered life, man must embrace this. I do not deny then, in regard to the knowledge and care of illnesses – to which those not following an ordered life frequently fall ill – that we have need of a doctor, with whom we should remain on good terms. Because if a friend is of great comfort simply by coming to visit and doing nothing more than to sympathize with you over your illness and to comfort you and to wish you well, how much more dear to you must the physician be, as your friend, who passes by to help you and promise you better health? But in conserving one's health, I believe we must embrace as our physician this ordered life, which – as shown – is a natural medicine of our very own,[*] [[truly much commended by the learned, and sought out (though under a different name) by many. Because the potable gold, or Elixir of Life, or whatever name it is called, what these overly curious investigators of things occult search for is none other than an ordered life, having the effect that is so desired by them. Because it conserves men – even those with a poor complexion – in good health, and lets them prosper to the age of one hundred years or more. And it does not let him end with illness, nor with any alteration of his humours, but rather out of the pure resolution of his radical moisture[32] that, by the end of life, is consumed. This and more is what many say gold, or an

---

[*] In 1591, a collected edition of Cornaro's treatise was published by his grandson Giacomo Alvise Cornaro Piscopia. According to Milani, the passage between double square brackets was revised by Giacomo Alvise, an alchemist (*Scritti ...*, p. 90).

32 The Galenic "lamp of life," the Stoic *callidum innatum,* or the natural heat of animals. "Life involved a continuous consumption of the body's 'innate heat' and 'radical moisture,' of which the latter served as fuel for the former (like the oil of a lamp, in a continually invoked metaphor)," N. Siraisi, *Clock and the Mirror ...*, p. 75; also see Robert Burton, *The Anatomy of Melancholy,* or see for example, N. Arikha, *Passions ....* The *radical moisture* refers to male semen, (*Sober ...*, p. 79n17, and see "Terminology": *Coitus,* and *Semen.*

Elixir, can do, which up to now many have searched for more often than they have experimented with. But let us be honest, men for the most part are highly sensual and unrestrained [*incontinenti*] and they would like to satisfy all their appetites and carry out an infinite number of disorders; and in order to do more of them, they wish to have a medicine with the principal virtue of dispelling illness, something that the wretched way of living they maintain lacks the power to introduce. Nevertheless, they put gold and other things through an alembic to recover it, and they do not see how it is the alembication of their brains[33] in their search of a medicine outside of Nature, which cannot have the effect they desire. While the one that is natural, which is readily at hand, they do not understand, or understanding it but because it does not delight their senses, it is not what they want.]]* And seeing that they cannot escape from crapula affecting them in a bad way at every stage, as an excuse they say it is better to live ten years less and satisfy oneself – without considering how important ten more years of life may be to a man and to a healthy life and a mature age, when men are known for what they are and what they know, and what they value in all manner of virtues; which cannot be at their perfection until that age. In regard to this – and without discussing the many others now – I will speak only of letters and the sciences in which the greater part of the beautiful and most celebrated books available to us were written when their authors were at this age and within those ten years left unappreciated by the *sensuali* so they can satisfy their appetites.[34] Be that as it may, I myself did not want to be like that; rather, I wanted to live these ten years, and if I had not done so I would not have written treatises that, my being alive and healthy over the past ten years, I have nevertheless written and that I know will be beneficial.

Furthermore, the aforementioned *sensuali* say that an ordered life is a life that cannot be lived. To which we respond that Galen, who was a truly great physician, lived it and deemed it the best medicine, as did Plato, Marcus Tullius, Socrates, and various other great men from times past, but so as not to be tedious I will not name them all. From our own era we have seen the great Pope Paulo [*sic*] Farnese practise it, and Cardinal Bembo, who thus lived a long life, and our two Dukes, Lando

---

33 *alembic … alembication of their brains*: apparatus or cap for a still … the distillation of their brains.

 * End of omitted passage. See above, asterisk note.

34 *sensuali*: see above, note 19. Cornaro refers to *sensuali* (brutes) as those who seek to satisfy only their sense driven appetites. Also see "Terminology," *s.v.*

and Donato,[35] and many others of lesser stature and those residing not only in the city but also the countryside, and that everywhere there is someone who benefits by following it. Therefore, having already done it and in any case with many practising it, a regulated life can be followed by anyone, all the more so because it does not require a great deal, rather, it involves nothing more than to begin, as the aforementioned Cicero [Tullius] and each of those practising it affirm. And because Plato, though he did live a regulated life, states in any event that a man of the Republic is unable to do so – having to suffer the heat, cold, and fatigue of various sorts, and other manner of things, which are all outside of an ordered life and are disorders – I respond that, as was said above, these are not the disorders that are important or that cause illness, or that make men die when the one so affected follows a sober life and not the two disorders of the mouth. A man of the Republic can well guard himself against [these two disorders], rather, it is necessary that he guard himself, because in so doing he cannot actually be exposed to those ills. Nor would he [living an ordered life] easily fall victim to them, making of those disorders what he is required to do, or even if exposed to them, being easily and quickly freed of them.

Here one could say to me, as some have, that whoever leads a regulated life – while always, being in good health, having eaten foods suitable for the infirm and in small quantities – has no need to remember anything else when ill. To this person, I would first say that Nature, who wishes to conserve man as long as she can, teaches us how we should care for ourselves when ill because she immediately takes appetite away from the ill, so they will not eat except for a little; because with this little, as was said before, she is content. Hence, the one who is ill, whether he led an ordered or disordered life up to that time, need only eat foods suitable to his illness, and these in even much less quantity than what he ordinarily would eat when healthy. For if he were to eat as much as usual, he would die from it, and if more, even sooner; because Nature – finding herself aggravated by illness – would be aggravated even more when given greater amounts of food than she could tolerate at that time. And

---

35 The following died at these approximate ages: Plato (428?–348? BCE) 76 years, Cicero (106–43 BCE) 63; Socrates (469–399 BCE) 70; Pope Paolo Farnese (1468–1549) 81; Pietro Bembo (1470–1547) 77; Pietro Lando (1462–1545) 83; Francesco (Donà) Donato (1468–1553) 85.

I would think this is enough for those ill to remember. Besides, we could better respond to them that whoever leads a regulated life cannot become ill, except on those rare occasions, and for so short a time, when he finds himself indisposed; because living regularly removes all the causes for illness, and with the causes removed its effect is removed. Therefore, whoever has followed an ordered life need not fear illness, since whoever is safe from its cause need not fear its effect.

An ordered life, then, is very advantageous and very virtuous and so beautiful and so blessed it should be followed and embraced by all, and even more so since it is not contrary to the way all sorts of men live. And it is easy to do, in that no one is required, while following it, to eat as little as I do, or not to eat fruit, fish and the other things that I do not eat. I eat little because that amount is enough for my small and weakened stomach; but fruit, fish, and those other foods do me harm, and so I leave them alone. The ones who benefit from those foods can, rather, they should, eat them, because those things are not forbidden to them. However, to them and to everyone else, eating as much as they want of the food they like is forbidden, since it is more than their stomach can digest, and the same is true for drinking. Therefore, the one for whom nothing is harmful, this person will only be subject to the rule of quantity not the quality of foods, which would be something extremely easy to do. Nor do I want anyone to say to me at this point that there are those who, living in a totally disordered way, arrive at the end of their days healthy and vigorous in the same way that more sober men do. I call this reasoning – being founded on what is doubtful – dangerous, and only very rarely occurs. And such an occurrence seems rather more miraculous than natural, which must not persuade us to live a disordered life, given that Nature has been overly generous to such persons; something that only a very few may hope to achieve. But whoever does not wish to believe these observations, being confident in his youth or strong complexion and perfect stomach, loses a great deal and is subjected everyday to illness and death. Therefore, I say it is more certain to live to be an old man, even with a poor complexion, for someone who follows a regulated and sober life, than the young man with a perfect complexion who lives a disorderly life. There is no doubt, however, that the one with a good nature can be conserved with order for more years than one whose nature is poor, and that God and Nature can operate in such a way that a man born with a perfect complexion may enjoy his health with few rules for living, over many years, and then die a very old man out of pure resolution,[36] as did the prosecutor Thomaso Contarini in Venice and the knight, Antonio Capo di Vacca in Padua.[37] But among one hundred thousand born, not even one can be found like them, so that those wanting to live for a long time in good health and to die without bother or trouble, out of resolution, must live regularly; for only in this way, and no other, are they able to enjoy the fruits of that life, which are almost infinite, and each to be infinitely appreciated. This is because – since it keeps the humours cleansed and benign in the body – [a sober life] does not then allow fumes from the stomach to ascend to the head;[38] so that the brain of the one who lives this way is always well cleansed, and he is always sound of mind. Hence, from considerations on the lowly and humble he ascends to the lofty and beautiful considerations on Divine things, to his utmost pleasure and contentment; because he thus considers and knows and understands what he never would have considered or known or understood, which is, how great the greatness of God is, and how great His Power, Wisdom, and Goodness. He then descends to Nature and understands that she is the daughter of this God, and sees and touches with his hand what at another age, or with a mind less clear, he would never have seen or touched. He then truly discerns the ugliness of vice, where in falls the man not knowing the way to curb human perturbations and the three troubling desires, which seem bred all three together within us to keep us always restless and tormented.

These three desires, for concupiscence, honours, and things, only increase in old persons lacking a regulated life. Because when they had passed their virile age, they left behind neither their senses nor appetites – as they should have – and to take in their place Continence and reason,

---

36 *Resolution* refers to the progressive decline of the organism, associated with the depletion of the body's radical moisture, *OED, s.v.*

37 Tommaso Contarini (1458–1554), prosecutor of San Marco, lived some ninety-six years. Antonio Capo di Vacca died in 1555 close to ninety years of age.

38 "[W]ine in excess added too greatly to the internal vital heat of digestion, totally subverting it, much as throwing too much wood on a fire suffocates it. This then leads to a corrupt 'concoction' in the stomach and the rising cloudy vapors that then surround the brain, making one dizzy, incoherent, and eventually julepated. It was in a sense, merely the mechanical force of fumes obfuscating the spirits coursing through the brain that caused drunkenness," K. Albala, *Banquet ...*, p. 106; or, "[b]ecause of their [beans, cabbage, etc.] indigestibility, these foods were thought literally to send fumes throughout the body, swelling it, or worse rising into the brain and causing nightmares. This wind could also enter the bloodstream and 'inflate' the extremities, the genitals included. This is one reason these foods were often considered aphrodisiacs," K. Albala, *Eating Right ...*, p. 59.

the virtues not left behind by one who lives an ordered life once past that age. The one, who, knowing such passions and such desires to be outside of reason, and having given himself completely over to [reason], has reflected on them, in addition to other vices, and in their place he moved closer to virtues and good works.[39] By these means, the wicked man he once was has made a good and honest life for himself, so that seeing himself reduced by old age to his resolution and to his end, knowing that by the sole Grace of God he had left vice behind, he was not afterwards a wicked man. And hoping as well that by the virtue of Jesus Christ Our Redeemer he would die in His Grace, he is not saddened by death, knowing that he must die, especially when laden with honours and fulfilled with life, he has attained that age to where many thousands of men born, living in a dissimilar way, merely arrive. And to an even greater extent he is not saddened, in that death does not arrive suddenly and unexpectedly with sharp and troubling changes to the humours, or with pain or fever, but with total calm and gentleness; because there is no cause for such an end in him if not for the lack of his radical moisture, which, as with a burning lamp, little by little disappears.[40] Thus he gently passes, free of illness, from this earthly and mortal life to that of a celestial and eternal one.

O blessed and truly happy life of order, may you be kept sacred and happy by men, just as the other – so very contrary to you – is wicked and unhappy; which can be clearly seen in the effects of one and the other. Even if men should know you only by saying that word aloud, your beautiful name, that beautiful name and beautiful sound is to say *ordered life* and *sobriety,* just as the ugly contrary thing is to say *disordered life* and crapula; rather, between these words, there seems to be that same difference as between saying *Angel* and *Devil.* And here I have given the reasons as to why I abandoned crapula and gave myself entirely over to a sober life, the method I undertook to do so, and what became of me, and finally, the comforts and benefits it brings to the one who follows it.

Now, since certain sensual and unreasonable men say it is not good to live for a long time and that once past the age of sixty-five years we can

---

39 *virtues … works*: virtue in Italian is *virtù* (Greek, *aretē*), a term of varied meanings. Here it is closer to manly qualities; manly excellence, manliness, courage, valour. Also see "Terminology": *virtue.*

40 On the metaphor of the lamp, see above, note 32. Also see Anton Maria Graziani on Cornaro's dying, "Intro.," p. 43n73.

no longer call it a life alive but a life dead – because they greatly fool themselves, as I will demonstrate (my hope being that each will attempt to reach my age so they may yet enjoy the most beautiful age of all) – I wish to recount at this time the things that amuse me now, and the enthusiasm I have at this stage of my life. It will assure everyone that it will be the same for each person who knows me, that is, the life I now live is completely alive and not dead; hence, [life] will be happy for many, with the very happiness we can have in this world. And they will have proof of this beforehand, because they see my prosperity – and not without the greatest admiration – in the way I can mount a horse on my own without need of assistance, climb not only stairs energetically on foot but an entire hillside, and how cheerful, pleasant, and content I am, freed of any perturbations of the soul and of any troubling thoughts; and in their place, joy and peace residing always in my heart, never to leave.

Moreover, they know how I pass my time, so that I do not regret my life, because I can only pass every hour of it in complete delight and pleasure. And quite often I have the privilege of conversing with many honourable Gentlemen – of great intellect and of breeding – being well read and excellent in other virtues. And when I lack their conversation, I take up a good book, and when I have read enough, I write, trying in this, and any other possible way, to help others as long as my strength permits. These are all things I do in the greatest of comfort, taking time with them while at my residence, which – aside from being in the most beautiful part of this noble and learned city of Padua – truly is still beautiful and praiseworthy, and of the kind no longer being constructed today. In one room I take refuge from the heat, in another from the cold, since I had them built according to architectural principles, which teach us how to do it. I also enjoy my various gardens, with their flowing streams alongside them, where I always find something delightful to do.

Another of my diversions is to go for several days in April and May, and again in September and October, to visit and enjoy my property in the hills of these Euganean Hills,[41] and in the most beautiful setting among them, with its fountains and gardens, and above all my beautiful and

---

41 Possible reference to the town of Fosson. The Euganean Hills, located just south of Padua, were praised by Petrarch (1304–1374), who resided at Arquà, and by Percy Bysshe Shelley (1792–1822) in his "Lines Written Among the Euganean Hills" (1818). Today called the "Tuscany of Venice," as wine producers are located in those Colli Euganei.

comfortable residence – where I occasionally go to hunt game suitable to my age – that is so accommodating and pleasant. I also enjoy time at my villa in the flatlands, which are very beautiful, with their lovely streets all leading to a beautiful piazza – in the midst of which there is the church, located in accordance to a position of high honour – made even more so as it is divided by a wide and flowing stream that is part of the Brenta River. On both sides of the river the town expands in territory, all composed of fertile and well-cultivated fields, which is still, by God's Grace, quite well inhabited, although this was not always so, rather the complete opposite, because it was full of swamps and foul air,[42] a tract of land more befitting water-snakes than men. But once I had the waters drained, the air then improved and people returned there to live; to the point where the number of souls multiplied many times over and made it the perfect place it is today. On this, in all truth, I can say that here in this place, I provided an altar to God, and a temple, and the souls to adore Him. They are all things that give me infinite pleasure, amusement, and happiness, every hour that I return there to see and enjoy them.

Each year during the same period, I revisit a few of the surrounding towns, and while enjoying my friends who live there, I take pleasure in discussing events and spending time with them. And through them I meet others from the area, men of fine intellect – architects, painters, sculptors, musicians and agriculturalists; in fact, men such as these, undoubtedly near our age, are fairly numerous. I see their latest works, their earlier ones, and always learn about things I am grateful to know. In their company I see the palaces, gardens, museum pieces, and the piazzas, churches, and fortresses; not overlooking anything that might be a source of pleasure or learning. But most of all, I enjoy the going and returning part of the trip, when I can reflect on the beauty of the places and lands while passing through them; those in the plains, those in the hillsides, close to rivers or fountains, with a range of beautiful dwellings and gardens surrounding them. Nor are these relaxations and pleasures any the less sweet and dear to me due to not being able to see well or to hear easily what is said to me, or because another of my senses may not be perfect, because they are all (by God's Grace) most perfect. This is

---

42 The village Cornaro saved is Codevigo (Codevico). See *Scritti* ..., p. 96n17. "Mal aria," the foul air from stagnant water, where mosquitoes breed, gave rise to the threat of malaria, and the belief at the time that miasma would result from the noxious fumes of the swamps.

especially true for my sense of taste, since I am able to taste even more now the simple food I eat wherever I go, unlike the way I once tasted during the time of my disordered life eating those many delicacies. Nor does it disturb me in any way to have to change beds, because I sleep well anywhere, and peacefully, without feeling disturbed by anything; and so while asleep my dreams are beautiful and pleasant. And it is with great pleasure and gratification that I see the success of an undertaking, very important to this State – I refer to the cultivation of lands left unutilized – which has since begun upon my proposal. It is something I never would have believed to see in my lifetime, knowing that undertakings of such great importance are slow in starting by Republics. However, I understood this and was there to meet with elected officials of this bureau for two months in a row, during the greatest heat of summer in these marshlands, nor did I ever feel bothered or fatigued or any other discomfort that I could have felt: so great is the power of an ordered life, which accompanies me no matter where I go. Furthermore, I am most hopeful and certain that I will see begun and finished another no less important undertaking, which is the conservation of our estuary, or lagoon, the remote and splendid fortress of my dear Homeland. This conservation was – and let it be said, not to make me feel good, but as the complete and honest truth – at my initiation, by my vigorously speaking out and diligently writing more than once to this Republic; for which, since I am naturally beholden to provide everything I can of comfort and benefit, I so dearly desire its long-lived happiness and conservation.

These are my real and important comforts. These are the relaxations and pastimes of my old age. A time more to be appreciated than the youth or old age of others, in that, being restored to health by God's Grace from the perturbations of the soul, and the infirmities of the body, [my old age] does not feel any of those contraries that miserably torment an infinite number of young people, and as many of the old and worn out, who are dispossessed of everything. And if to things great and important, it is admissible to compare the minor – or better, what is generally considered just a pastime – then, for me, included among the fruits of the sober life, is the fact that at the age of eighty-three I was able to compose a most agreeable comedy, full of genuine laughter and enjoyable witticisms. This style of poem is ordinarily the fruit of the youthful phase of man, just as tragedy is usually the effect of old age; the former being such for its charm and cheerfulness in relation to youth, as the latter is for its melancholy in growing old. Now, if that fine old gentleman,

Greek by nationality, and a poet,[43] was praised for having written a trag-edy at the age of seventy-three, and for this he was deemed to be healthy and energetic – with a tragedy being all of a mournful and melancholic poem – why should I be held as less fortunate and less healthy than he, being his elder by ten years, for having written a comedy that is a happy and pleasant composition of renown? Certainly, if I am a fair judge of myself, I would like to think that I am healthier and more cheerful at this age than he was in his life, being at the time some ten years younger than me.

And because there is no lack of entertainment, with my many years, which renders my age less regretful or my contentment no less bountiful, I see it almost as a kind of immortality in the succession of my descen-dants. Because upon returning home, I then find not one, or two, but eleven of my grandchildren, the eldest of whom is eighteen years old and the youngest being two; and all are the children of one father and one mother. They are all very healthy, [[all the most beautiful,]][44] and as far as we can now tell, all very proficient and dedicated to letters and well mannered. From among the younger children I always en-joy one or the other as my clown, because those little imps, from the ages of three to five, really are natural clowns; and the older ones re-main, in one way or another, companions to me. And because they have naturally perfect pitch, I also enjoy listening to them playing different in-struments and to their singing; rather, I myself sing along with them be-cause my voice has more clarity and is more sonorous than ever before. And when surrounded by such beautiful children, I am then likened by whoever sees me to a God the Father, encircled as in paintings by His Angels and Archangels.[45]

---

43 The reference is suggested to be Sophocles (497?–406? BCE) and his play, *Philoctetes,* though written some years earlier, it was performed for the first time in 409 BCE, when the tragedian was nearly 88 years old. In 1558, Cornaro was likely either seventy-four or seventy-six years old. See A. Cornaro, *Alvise Cornaro: La vita sobria.* A cura di Arnaldo Di Benedetto (Zingonia: TEA, [1993] 1997), p. 55n18.

44 *all the most beautiful:* this phrase was omitted by Cornaro's grandson (1591 edition). See "Intro.," p. 19.

45 *And when surrounded...Archangels:* a passage excised for its "almost blasphemous" tone, by Evangelista Oriente, a Paduan doctor and friend to Giacomo Alvise (Cornaro's grandson), who had asked Oriente to oversee changes to the *Vita sobria* for the 1591 collected edition. See "Intro.," p. 33. On the significance of Cornaro's voice, see *Eulogy,* p. 132n2.

These are the diversions of my old age. By which one sees that the life I live is a life alive and not dead, like those who know little about it say, and to whom, so it is clear how much I respect other ways of living, I say in truth that I would not exchange my life nor my age with any of the young who live following their appetites; even if he does has an excellent complexion, since I know first hand that such a person is subjected daily, rather every hour, to a thousand sorts, as I have said, of infirmities and death. In fact, this is so clearly evident that there is no need of any proof, as I also remember well what I did at that age. I know how much that age is one of being only inconsiderate, and how much the young, helped by their innate heat, are so bold and self assured in whatever they do and hope for the best in everything, whether it is because of their lack of past experience, or for the guarantee the young believe they have for living long into the future. And so they fearlessly risk every sort of danger to themselves, and with reason pushed aside and being left to decide on their own about their cravings, they try to satisfy every one of their appetites; not seeing, these poor wretches, that they are acquiring what they would not wish to have, which is infirmity – as I have so stated many times – and death. Of these two evils, the one is a serious and troublesome thing to suffer, the other completely unbearable and frightening. It is unbearable to those who let themselves be prey to their senses – especially to the young, who, it seems, die from too much damage before their time – and frightening to those who think about the errors that fill our mortal lives, and about the revenge that only the Justice of God can take in the eternal punishment of the sinner.

Upon encountering my present age (always by God's Grace), I find myself free from one and the other of these torments. From the one, because I am sure and certain that I cannot become ill, having removed any cause for illness with my sacred medicine; and from the other, which is that of death, because of the habit by now learned so many years ago to yield to reason. Thus, not only does it seem an ugly thing to fear what one cannot escape, but I am still hoping, when I arrive at that moment, to take some consolation from the Grace of Jesus Christ. What is more, though I know very well that like everyone else my life must come to an end, this end, however, is still so far away that I cannot make it out. Because I know I will not die if not out of pure resolution, having already, with my regulated form of living, closed off all other pathways to death and blocked the means for humours in my body to wage war; other than what all the elements, having combined together at my birth, can wage against me.[46] For I am not so foolish not to see, in the fact that I was born, that it is proper for me to die; yet the beautiful and desirable death is the one Nature provides us through resolution. Indeed, it is because Nature, having been the one to form our bond to life, finds an easier way to undo that bond and to delay undoing it until later and thus avoid the violence of infirmities [disorders]. It is that death, dispensing with the poetic, which can [truly] be called death, for at that moment it is not life, which cannot be anything else. This does not occur until after the interval of a very old age, and the unavoidable result of great weakness; because little by little, and over a long time, men are reduced in terms of no longer being able to walk, and barely to reason, becoming blind, deaf, and curved over, and filled with every other ill. But I can still be certain (by the Grace of God) of being far from such an end, rather, I do believe that my own soul – which has so good a home in my body, finding nothing but peace, love, and harmony, not only among its humours but even among the senses and reason – enjoys being there and is most content; so it is reasonable that it will take a great deal of time and the force of many years to make it leave. It certainly can be concluded, therefore, that I will live for many years in health and prosperity, revelling in this beautiful world; beautiful for the one who knows how to make it beautiful for himself, as I have done, hoping to be able to do the same through the Grace of God even into the next. And it is all by means of virtue and a blessed regulated life, which I undertook by becoming a friend of reason and an enemy of the senses and appetites, something easily done by anyone who wishes to live in the way befitting a man.

Now, if this life of sobriety is so happy, if its name is so charming and delightful, if its possession so easy, and conservation so firm and assured, no other duty remains to me except to pray (since I cannot achieve my wish through the oratory of persuasion), that each man, good of heart and rational of speech, embrace this the richest treasure of life. And since it surpasses all other riches and goods in this world (bringing us a long and healthy life), it is thus worthy of always being loved, pursued, and conserved by each of us. This is that very divine Sobriety,

---

46 According to classical thought, when we are born, the elements and humours ideally are proportionally balanced (*eukrasia*). Disproportional humours (*dyskrasia*) can produce physical and mental illness. See "Intro.," p. 20, and see above, note 35. And see, for example, N. Siraisi, *Medieval* ..., p. 105, or N. Arikha, *Passions* ... . Also see "Terminology": *Element, Humours.*

favoured by God, friend to Nature, daughter of Reason, sister of all Virtues, companion to Temperate Living; modest, kind, content with little, and regulated and distinguished in its operations. From it grows – as from a root – life, health, happiness, industry, learning, and all deeds proper to every well-born and self-composed soul [*animo*]. Divine and human laws favour it. From it flee, as so many clouds from the sun, repletions,[47] disorders, gluttonies, damaging humours, distempers, fevers, pains, and threats of death. Its beauty charms every noble heart. Its certainty assures each person graceful and enduring conservation. Its ease invites everyone to experience its victories with little inconvenience. And finally, it promises to be a grateful and benign custodian of life, as much for the rich as for the poor, as much for men as for women, as much for the old as for the young; as the one that teaches to the rich decency, to the poor frugality, to men Continence, to women modesty, to the old a defence from death, to the young the hope of a stable and secure life. Sobriety sees that our senses are purified, our body light, our intellect lively, our spirit happy, our memory holds, our motions quick, and our actions ready and able. In sobriety, the soul – almost relieved of its earthly weight – experiences a great part of its liberation: spirits lightly move through arteries, blood runs through veins,[48] a temperate and gentle heat has a gentle and temperate effect; and finally, these powers of ours, serve, through the most beautiful order, a cheerful and agreeable harmony.

O most blessed and most innocent Sobriety, the only refuge of Nature, benign Mother of human life, as true a medicine for our spirit [*animo*] as for our body, how men should praise and thank you for your gracious gifts! You provide them with a way to conserve that very good – life I mean – and health; and God did not want us to have greater feelings for anything but it in this world, life and existence being what is naturally so greatly appreciated by every living being, and willingly safeguarded.

---

47 *Repletion*: the condition resulting from consuming excessive food or drink (versus depletion), linked to vascular congestion; and a "surfeit, a full plethoric condition or habit of body," *OED, s.v.*

48 How the blood circulated was not well understood at the time, as Cornaro "still believed, after Galen, that blood passing through the liver, heart and brain filled up with the three fundamental spirits of the human body: the natural, vital and animal," *Scritti ...,* p. 101n24. William Harvey (1578–1657) will further refine knowledge of blood in his *Exercitatio Anatomica de Motu Cordis et Sanguinis in Animalibus* (1628).

However, because I do not now intend to compose a panegyric of this rare and excellent Sobriety, I will finish here, remaining sober for this part: not because there is not an infinite number of things still to be recounted on it, beyond what has already been said, but so I may return to the rest of its merits at a more opportune time.

(1558)

Addition* to the Treatise on the Sober Life by Messer Alvise Cornaro

I wrote my Treatise on the Sober Life in the hope and desire of helping many others, knowing from experience that it conserves a man's health and gives him long life, and is something easily maintained; because if it were difficult to do I could not have followed it, since I am but a man. Nor, however, have I yet heard that others have adopted this way of life. And though it is praised by all, it was nonetheless avoided by all, almost abhorred, as if it were depraved and not the daughter of blessed and virtuous Continence, born of Divine Reason; a special grace conceded to man by Our Lord so that he may be different and superior to brute animals. But because I would like to help and to keep my companions, I still wanted to write this brief paper in which I will deal especially with the elderly, who ordinarily suffer all the time – some with the pain of gout, of their side, or catarrh, and of other similar illnesses deemed as incurable – hoping that at least these, to free themselves of those [ills], would make themselves my companions and attempt to become healthy, in the way I have done. I, who was overcome with said ills as the result of the disordered life I led, and of my poor complexion, and of my bad stomach – from which no good conditions are generated – was thus full of illnesses that doctors were unable to relieve with their medicine or their bath waters, or any of their other very potent and invigorating treatments. Yet I resolved it simply with the one diet, and with the regulated order of eating and drinking. For I understood clearly enough that my infirmities

---

* Prior to Milani's critical edition (1983), Cornaro's *Aggionta* or "Addition" had never appeared in any *Vita sobria* edition, not even in that of his grandson's of 1591. The "Addition" appears here for the first time in an edition in English.

had originated from my over eating, and from eating all sorts of different foods that were contrary to my stomach and which had brought me to extreme repletion; and in truth this is what caused those said ills. Many of the elderly referred to above can yet attest this, for which they – being themselves assailed by these ills – adopt the diet, using neither doctors nor other medicines and through diet alone free themselves; because against the repletion that generates illness there is not a more appropriate medicine than the diet. Being then the diet completely opposite to repletion, and with illness removed by the diet alone, it need be said that illness proceeds only from repletion. If from diet alone we can be free of ills, there is no doubt that with the illness removed, whoever continues to follow the diet (yet not so strictly as when he was ill, but instead a moderate diet, which is characteristic of the sober life) will conserve his health. Because its virtue is less in conserving someone who has recovered his health, than it is in its virtue to free him of the illness that actually afflicts him, the illness (as I have said) that comes from repletion. However, men who are accustomed to different foods and in excessive amounts, hoping that eating a great deal conserves them better than eating a little – led by their senses and voracious gluttonous appetite – while thinking they are conserving themselves, they are killing themselves before their time. Even at such an advanced age, when reason assumes its place – and in older men it should have subdued their senses – they should therefore understand that since they have grown old, so too their stomachs, which are unable to digest as much food now as they once were able when young. And they should know this: that a little food can be digested by the stomach, not a lot of food, being that a lot is harmful, since a little is beneficial. Furthermore, they should understand that the old need little food to conserve their life and health, since Nature is content with little, and that a large amount of food, because it cannot be digested by them, converts into repletion, which [repletion] generates ill humours and ill humours generate infirmities; and what I say can actually be observed and it cannot be denied. Nor do they deny it, but they excuse themselves by saying they cannot live on a small amount of plain food – which is all that is necessary for a sober life – because it would never appeal to their taste, and therefore, not enjoying it, they would fall into mortal weakness. To this, I respond and say that if their taste is not for natural foods, it comes from the fact that because of disorders their taste has become disordered, and its natural order [balance] has been taken away. It would return to its proper nature if they were to try the diet for four or six days, because then, together with a great desire to eat, they would taste more of plain and pure bread than what they do not taste now of their many different foods. And since it is a true and natural thing, which everyone knows and accepts, we must conclude that good taste [palate] comes from eating little; and with this little, the humours are perfected and conserve health and with health a long life. In order to help them, then, let us suppose that their taste is less for simple foods than for combined and different foods. It is not, therefore, that old men should instead suffer the ills that their gluttony makes them suffer, given their understanding that ills and pains last longer while the pleasure of gluttony is less than brief; that is, the moment it begins it is over. Thus, [gluttony] should be little appreciated, whereas our health should be appreciated a great deal; because from health follows long life, from gluttony violent dissolution. But in response to those, who – though admitting that a sober life conserves man's health – nevertheless deny that it can prolong life, which (as they say) is determined for man at his birth and has a preset end, I say they should not judge that end to be absolutely determined, but rather – since it is [in fact] their death – to be the resolution of the regulated [body] as prescribed by the Divine Mind. A prescription that does not necessarily operate, however, and just as predestination is conditioned – as the Holy Scriptures teach – so too this end is conditional.[49] Do we not have the example (as I recall having read in the Book of Kings) that the Just and Immutable Lord prolonged the life of Hezekiah by fifteen years?[50] I myself can attest this and I am sure that if I had not faithfully followed the diet and a sober life, I would have been dead long ago, just as the doctors confirmed when they had given up on me without having found a way to liberate me of my illness. But let us suppose that this [end] is not prolonged. We can even say – at least in order to live healthy for the time conceded to us – that we should not be bound to it very much, careful that to live healthy is the truest idea of life and to live infirm is under the most horrible shadow of death, where I myself did not wish to live. And yet, I truly live life (albeit not an absolute and eternal one, which we do not have in this world) at this age of

---

49 Cornaro was not the first to discuss the possibility of a long life, but he was the first to advise that in following the sober life, longevity could be attained by every man, no matter his age, complexion, condition, social or economic status.

50 "And I will add to your days fifteen years. I will deliver you and this city from the hand of king of Assyria; and I will defend this city for My own sake and for the sake of My servant David": II Kings 20: 6, *NKJV.*

eighty-five years.[51] My life is filled with happiness, contentment and every good, always speaking, however, of the good that this frail and mortal life can offer us; nor do my senses lack their usual power, nor my body prosperity, nor has my memory diminished, nor has my heart lost its usual vigour. Rather, my thoughts [*cervello*] are always serene with the acumen of an intelligence unoccupied by contrary humours, nor am I tempted by uncontrolled senses, nor have I wasted away because of moderate abstinence; my teeth are strong, my voice still harmonious with a well disposed tone, nor is it hindered by any sort of catarrh, nor have my legs lost their ability to climb steep stairs. But more than this I would say that neither the accidents of the soul nor its passions nor its perturbations trouble me; not even the thought of death, because I am certain I have removed, by means of a sober life, the circumstances that produce illness and an unnatural death, and I call it [unnatural] because kind Mother Nature does not care for so violent an act [*moto*]; though some said [death] is Terrible, they were not considering, as do the Ethnics,[52] that it is the path to immortality. I thus conclude that mine will not be death (not wanting to overlook the opinion of Dionysius)[53] but the separation of these two junctures, from which will come pure resolution, from which can be seen from the said benefits and indications that I am a long

---

51 Depending on his birth date, 1482 (Milani) or 1484 (Menegazzo), Cornaro is either seventy-seven or seventy-nine years of age in 1559, *Scritti ...*, pp. 139–41. Emilio Menegazzo, after having analyzed the relevant documents, deduced among other things that Cornaro was born in 1484, and that he had written his own eulogy; see "Intro.," p. 40n65. According to Milani, in his 1966 work "Altre osservazioni ...," Menegazzo possibly errs in regard to Cornaro's age by two years in reference to his eulogy (see "Intro.," p. 45n76).

52 *Ethnic*: Heathens, polytheistic and pleasure-seeking. It is a term "applied to persons or races whose religion is neither Christian, or Jewish, nor Muslim." Known also as pagans, or Gentiles, *ethnic* "applied also to Muslims; but in modern usage, for the most part, restricted to those holding polytheistic beliefs," *OED, s.v.*

53 Reference to psuedo-Dionysius (late 400s or early 500s CE?), the unknown Christian author of *Corpus* Areopagiticum. It was with his works, "translated from Greek into Latin in the ninth century, [that] Western medieval thinkers inherited the notion of 'negative theology.' This meant that we human beings in our finiteness could never adequately know God, in his infinite majesty. But we could at least approach him through saying what he was not" Christopher S. Celenza, "The revival of Platonic Philosophy" in *The Cambridge Companion to Renaissance Philosophy*, ed. James Hankins (Cambridge: University of Cambridge Press, 2007), p. 74. Cf. Dionysius the Areopagite (650–725 CE), who was incorrectly attributed to be the author of these thoughts.

way from death. Resolution will therefore come to those who maintain a sober life, which is easy to do, for the reasons I have demonstrated and for the experience that can be seen in me, a mere man. And I affirm that a sober life is a cheerful and enjoyable one to implement; hence, I would neither write nor reason so heartily on it if not for my great desire to be helpful.

(1559/60)

A Brief Compendium of The Sober Life by Alvise Cornaro With Many Things Added, Especially Useful and Necessary for Those Who Are Old

My Treatise on the Sober Life, as I had hoped, has begun to help those born with a poor complexion, while with each episode and every little disorder they have owing to their weak complexion, they feel so indisposed they could not possibly feel worse; something that cannot really happen to those born with a good complexion. And so in order to live healthy, those with a bad one, having read my Treatise, have adopted the [sober] life, reassured how beneficial it is by my experience. For this reason, I would like to help those born with a good complexion, because in using it as their foundation they are living a disordered life; thus, as they near sixty years of age or thereabouts, they are afflicted with various ills and pains – some of them with gout, some in their side, some in their stomach, and other similar ills – none of which they would have [suffered] had they adopted a sober life. And seeing as they die of them before arriving at eighty years, they would have lived to one hundred, the end conceded by God and by our own Mother Nature to us her sons. We can believe that she would want each of us to reach that end so as to enjoy life at every age, but because our birth is subject to the revolutions of the Heavens, which have great power at our birth – with their greatest power over good or poor complexions – it is something that Nature cannot foresee; for if she were able to do so, she would see to it that everyone was born with a good one. But she hopes that, having been born with intelligence and reason, man on his own, together with art, is able to compensate for whatever the Heavens have taken from him, and through the art of a sober life, to understand the way to free himself of a poor complexion, and live a long life always in good health. Because there is no doubt that man, by means of art, is partially able to free himself from the predispositions of the Heavens, being common knowledge that the Heavens predispose but do not compel [us]; and so the learned have said that a wise man governs the stars.[54]

I was born very choleric, so much so that no one could be around me, and I learned and saw in myself that a choleric person is demented at the time – I refer to when ruled by his choler – because neither he nor his thinking [*intelletto*] is reasonable. And I resolved to free myself of choler by being reasonable, so that now, though born choleric, I do not behave with such an attitude except to a certain extent. Similarly, one born with a poor complexion can, through reason and a sober life, live healthy over a long time, as I have done. And my being born with a very poor complexion made it almost impossible that I would live past the age of forty years, and now at the age of eighty-six I find myself healthy and prosperous.[55] And if it were not for the fact that during my long and extreme illnesses – many of them occurring in my youth when the doctors had given up on me, and a large part of my radical moisture was removed, which can never be restored – I would hope to arrive at said end. But I know that, reasonably, it will be an impossibility, but on this – as I will demonstrate – I do not dwell, as it is quite enough for me to have lived forty-six years longer than I should have, and that during such an old age all my sensory capacities [*sentimenti*] are at their perfection; even my teeth, my voice, my memory, and my heart, but above all my brain functions more than it ever has, nor have these things diminished in capacity with the passing of the years. It is because I continue to grow from the order of a sober life, by which, seeing that my years are increasing, I therefore decrease the quantity of food I eat, since such a decrease is necessary; nor can one do otherwise given that we cannot live forever. And nearer to the end of his life, man is reduced no longer to eating but to drinking, with some difficulty, one egg yolk everyday and to finish [life] through resolution, free of pain or illness, as I will be, and this is

54 *Vir sapiens dominabitur astris,* often translated as the suggestive "a wise man will rule the stars," is attributed to Ptolemy (Claudius Ptolemaeus) (90/100–c.170), possibly of Greek or Egyptian origin, who was a mathematician, geographer, and astronomer, astrologer, as well as a theorist on optics and music. He is famously known for his study on astronomy, *Almagest* (150? CE).

    Stars also signify the planets, hence astrology.

55 In 1561 Cornaro is either seventy-seven or seventy-nine years of age.

very important.[56] [Resolution] will happen for everyone who follows a sober life, no matter what or to what extent his condition is, whether it is a major or middling or minor condition, because we are each the product of only one species and of the four elements. And since living healthy and long should be greatly appreciated by man, as I will discuss, I conclude that he is obliged to do whatever work he can in order to live, and that he should not commit to live for a long time without the means of a sober life. Because he may have heard that some live – without following that life – up to the age of one hundred years, always in good health, by eating large amounts of any kind of food and drinking any wine, and therefore promise that it will be the same for him. But in doing so, he commits two errors: first, that out of a hundred thousand born, not one such person can be found; and second, that such persons become ill and die ill, and can never be assured of dying without ills and infirmity. Therefore, the only certain way and life to live, at least once past the age of forty years, is to adopt a sober life – which is not difficult to follow – in the company of the many we have read about who have followed it in the past and the many who now follow it as I do. And given that we are men, then as a man, being a reasonable animal, he can do as much as he wants to do.

This [[sober]] life only consists of the following two things: quantity and quality.[57] The first, quality, consists simply of not eating foods or drinking wines contrary to one's stomach; quantity consists of not eating or drinking except the amount the stomach can easily digest. That quantity and that quality, however, should be understood by the time a man

---

56 "Containing all four elements in proportion ... Eggs, therefore, provide perfect nourishment for people of all ages, complexions, and in all seasons," K. Albala, *Eating Right ...*, pp. 76–7.

In Christianity, the representation of an egg also signifies birth, rebirth, and the cosmos.

57 Milani writes: "The rule of quantity and of quality is not an invention of Cornaro. It goes back to Galen, [with whose work] besides, Cornaro proves to be quite familiar; but the physician of antiquity only recommended it for the elderly ... We see that the alimentary prescriptions of Galen are very similar to those that Cornaro adopts; but what surprises is the extraordinary work of reduction to the simple elementary rule of *quantity-quality* that Cornaro succeeded in making out of the teachings of the classical maestro." See "Intro.," pp. 26–8. Cf. Alcmaeon's theory on suitability and quantity of food.

reaches forty, fifty, or sixty years of age, and whoever maintains these two orders, lives an ordered and sober life, which has so much virtue and power that within that body, the humours are perfected, balanced, and integrated. Thus made good, the humours cannot be activated nor altered by any other disorders the body may have – suffering the cold and heat, being over tired, fasting, and others – if they are not too extreme. In which case, the body, unable to maintain the two orders of the mouth, prompts its humours to alter and to cause fever, so causing him to die before his time. Man is therefore obliged to maintain these orders [of quantity and quality], it being a certainty that whoever does not maintain them, either because of those said disorders or for the various and infinite other ones, he will always risk illness and death from each of these [disorders], since he lives a disordered and not a sober life.

It is quite true even for those who maintain the two [orders] of the mouth, which is the sober life, that for each of the other disorders experienced they feel them for one or two days, but without fever. Thus, they still feel the revolutions of the Heavens, but neither the Heavens nor those disorders can induce the alteration of the humours of one who maintains a sober life; and this is reasonable and natural, because the two disorders of the mouth are internal and the others are external. But because there are those elderly, being especially sensual, who say neither the quantity or quality of foods or wines harm them, they then eat and drink a great deal of everything; and because they do not know where in the body their stomach is, it is certain they are still abnormally sensual and friends of gluttony. Our response to them is that what they claim cannot be natural, because it necessitates that when one is born, he be born with a complexion that is hot or cold or temperate, and that hot foods benefit hot complexions and cold foods the cold and combined foods the temperate: something which is not possible in nature. The especially sensual ones, as those above, cannot even say they do not become ill from time to time and are then freed by voiding themselves with medicine and a strict diet; from which we understand that their illness comes from the repletion of too much food and of foods contrary to their stomachs.

There are still other old men who say it is necessary for them to eat and drink a great deal to sustain their natural body heat, which is decreasing as their years increase, and that they are compelled to eat a great deal, and of the foods appealing to their taste for the hot or cold or temperate; and if they had to live a sober life, they would rather die. We respond that our own Mother Nature – so that her elderly could conserve themselves – has seen to it that they are able to live on little food, as I am doing; because a large amount cannot be digested by the stomach of an old person, it too having become old and weak. Thus, he need not fear dying from eating little, if by so little, when he is ill, he frees himself; because so little is that part of the diet by which he regains his health. And if, with this little, he regains his health and is restored, how can he doubt that by eating a larger quantity – that larger quantity of a sober life – he would not stay alive and be healthy?

Others say it is better to suffer three or four times a year their usual ills – gout, their sides, or other ills – than to suffer the entire year unable to satisfy their appetite for eating everything that tastes better to them, since they are certain that with the medicine of simple dieting they can be free of those ills. The response is that with increasing years comes decreasing natural body heat, and that dieting does not always have the same amount of virtue as the disorder of repletion has force; and so they are compelled to die of these very ills, because [disorders] shorten life, just as health conserves it.

Others say it is better to live ten years less rather than not satisfy one's appetite. To them we respond that a long life should be very much appreciated by men of fine intellect, but as for the others, there is little harm done if they do not appreciate it, because they make the world ugly and it is not a bad thing if they were to die.[58] But it is bad if those of fine intellect were to die, because if he is a cardinal, once past eighty years he becomes Pope; if from the Republic, a leader; if from letters, he is thought of as a god on earth; and likewise for those in all other professions.

---

58 Speculation over whom Cornaro would heap this criticism may possibly lead to the notorious Pietro Aretino (1492–1556) ("Intro.," p. 59), who openly opposed a sober life ("Immortality ...," p. 189n9). The Tuscan dramatist, poet, first modern *poligrafo* (journalist), and the satirist feared by popes and everyone was placed in the great poem *Orlando furioso* by Ludovico Ariosto (1474–1533) as "*il flagello de' principi, il divin Pietro Aretino*," immortalizing the divine Aretino's known reputation as the "scourge of princes." He is regarded as the first writer of modern literary pornography: *I ragionamenti* (1534–1536), for example, or the earlier *I Modi* (1524–1527) with their *Sonetti lussuriosi*: "lascivious" sonnets written to accompany the explicit engravings published by Marcantonio Raimondi (1480–1534) that were based on the erotic paintings of Giulio (Pippi) Romano (1499–1546). Cornaro, formulating his thoughts on a sober life over many years – letter to Commander Aluvise Cornaro, or to Speroni (*Sober ...*, p. 6, p. 155) – only published the "Compendium" in 1561, after Aretino had been deceased and his works placed by Pope Paul IV on the Vatican's 1558/9 Index Librorum Prohibitorum (Prohibited Books), and ordered burned.

[[Still others remain such enemies of the sober life that they devote themselves to finding a medicine so perfect that enables them to live a disordered life, and to be free of illness with that [medicine]. They find certain alchemists who promise to make them the medicine they desire, either that of potable gold or that other, *Eliser vitae*: medicines, which, so they say, keep a man young and healthy in his old age. And in believing them – because they want to – by such [medicines] they are killing themselves, without regard to the cost, and without considering that if those medicines had such great virtue, the upper class would be making use of them, and they would also have been used in the past by our many great emperors. But such alchemists were never found to have succeeded in their ways and methods not found in Nature. And we know that a natural and true medicine, like the diet and life of sobriety, cannot keep an old man who is in his dotage as anything but old, not young – so how is it then possible that by means of an artificial art he could be made young?]][59]

There are others, who, when they reach that age – even though their stomach naturally becomes less able to digest – still do not want to decrease their food, but to increase it instead. And because by eating twice a day they cannot digest much quantity, they resolve to eat only once a day, to allow the long interval between one meal and the next to operate, and so be able to eat as much food at one time as the same amount they would have eaten in two meals; thereby eating an equal amount. But their stomachs, loaded with so much food, begin to suffer and go bad and to change that surplus food into bad humours; and these are what kill a man before his time. I have never met even one person to take up that life who lived for a long time. But they might possibly live, if, as their years increase, they were to decrease the quantity of food and eat more

---

59 Giacomo Alvise Cornaro Piscopia (1539–1608), Cornaro's first born grandson, and an alchemist, had this passage (between square brackets) excised, see *Scritti ...*, pp. 110–11n5. Giacomo Alvise and his brother Marcantonio were avid supporters of the alchemist Marco Bragadin (Mamugnà), the "Cypriot," but in reality a swindler who claimed he could turn mercury into gold. He came under investigation by the Venetian Senate and by the Inquisition after stealing from the Franciscan Order hosting him; whence he escaped to France. In 1589, about to be captured in Italy, he fled to Munich, where he was at first well received by the Duke, but with evidence mounting against him, Bragadin was forced to confess to his fakery. He was eventually tried and decapitated in 1591. See "Intro.," pp. 34–6; also see, Horatio F. Brown, *Venetian Studies.* (London: Elibron Classics Series, Adamant Media Corporation's facsimile reprint of Kegan Paul, Trench & Co., London, 1887, 2004), pp. 259–90.

times throughout the day – but a little at a time. Because an old stomach cannot digest a large quantity, only a little; and so the old man returns to eating like a young boy who eats many times a day.

Others say that a sober life may well conserve a man's health, but it cannot prolong his life. We respond that we know who prolonged his life in the past, and we know that I prolong it now. It cannot then be said that a sober life shortens it, since infirmity shortens it; and so there is no doubt that this does not shorten life. It is thus better to live being healthy at all times than to live being ill many times, in order to conserve one's radical humour; by which we can reasonably conclude that a sacred Sober Life may be the true Mother of health and long life.

O venerable Sober Life, so beneficial to man, helping him as much as you do allows him to live long, and by living to an old age he becomes so reasonable that through reason he frees himself of the bitter fruit of sensuality – the enemy of reason, which [reason] is proper to man – and these bitter fruits are his passions and perturbations. Furthermore, you also free him of the horrendous thought of death! And I, your good disciple, am much obliged to you, for because of you I enjoy this beautiful world, which truly is beautiful for the one who knows the way to make it so, through your means, as I knew to do for myself! Nor at any other age – when I was young and only sensual and living my disordered life – could I ever have made it as beautiful for myself. Even though, in order to enjoy [life] at each age, I did not save on expenses or anything else, I found that each pleasure at each of those ages had its contraries; and so I never knew the world was beautiful until I arrived at this age. O truly happy life that, other than the blessings (as named before) you grant to your old, to be kind you reduce his stomach and so perfectly that he enjoys plain bread more than the greatest delicacies he had once enjoyed in his youth. This operates because you are reasonable, knowing that bread is the most fitting food for man when accompanied by a desire to eat. And with a sober life, he will always have this natural companion,

---

Marco Bragadin is not to be confused with the martyred Marc Antonio Bragadin (1523–1571), a Venetian national hero and military captain (Mamugnà falsely claimed to be his son) who, at the infamous battle at Famagusta (Cyprus), was first tortured "then flayed alive, and his skin stuffed with straw, was paraded through the streets under a red umbrella. The trophy [the body] was taken to Constantinople, but was stolen from the arsenal there in 1580, and is now contained in an urn in the Church of SS. Giovanni e Paolo in Venice." Horatio F. Brown, *Life on the Lagoons* (London: Rivingtons, 1909), pp. 57–8.

because by always eating so little, the stomach – by containing little – will always have a desire to eat, up to the end; which is why he enjoys plain bread so much. I know this from my own experience, and I can say that I enjoy it so much that I fear I could stray into the vice of gluttony, if not for the fact that I know eating is but a necessity, and that we cannot eat a more natural food.[60]

And you, Mother Nature, so loving of your old that to conserve him longer, you gave him the means of doing so by eating little. And to favour and benefit him more in this, you demonstrate to him that, since in his youth he ate twice a day, in his old age he should divide that daily food of two meals into four, because that food, so divided, will be more easily digested by his stomach. And, because as a young man he ate only twice a day, in old age he should eat four times a day, and continue to decrease the quantity as his years continue to increase. This is what I observe, since you demonstrate it to me, and therefore my spirits, which are not oppressed by a large amount of food but only sustained, are always happy. And [your] virtue is best shown following a meal, for I am compelled, after eating, to sing and then to write, nor does my writing after eating harm me, nor has my intellect ever been as good as it is now; nor am I drowsy after eating, because a little amount of food cannot send fumes from my stomach up to my head.[61]

How very beneficial it is for someone old to eat so little! Knowing this, I eat only enough for me to live on – and these are my foods: first, bread, *panatella*[62] or broth with an egg or other similar good soups; for meat I eat veal, kid, and beef; I eat any sort of poultry, I eat partridge, and fowl such as thrush; I also eat fish, saltwater ones like sea-bream or similar, and from freshwater, pike and the like. These are all foods suitable for the old, and they must be content with these, not wanting more, since they are ample; and the old man who out of poverty cannot have these foods, is able to conserve himself on bread, *panatella*, and eggs. And in truth, someone poor will not be left wanting, unless he is a beggar, or

---

60 One of Cornaro's odes to bread is found in a letter to Speroni (*Sober ...*, p. 161). The word for bread itself, K. Albala recalls, affects us in other ways as "even the words *accompany* and *companion* derive from the Latin words to share bread [*pane*]," in *Food in Early ...*, p. 22.

61 See above, note 38.

62 *Panatella* is a light soup traditionally recommended for the sick (Alcmaeon, Galen), made of stale bread combined with water, or milk, or broth. Variations of it may include an egg for thickening, or other ingredients. Also see "Terminology," *s.v.*

what is called a beggar – but we must not think about that one, because
he came to this [circumstance] out of his ineptitude and is better dead
than alive because he makes the world ugly.[63] But if the poor cannot eat
well on bread or *panatella* or eggs, they need only eat the quantity they
can digest; and the one observing quantity and quality cannot die, unless
from pure resolution without any illness.

What a difference there is from a life of order to one of disorder: the
one lets you live healthy and for a long time, the other lets you live with
infirmities and die before your time; by which it is understood that the
disordered life is an unhappy one. O unhappy and miserable life, my
enemy, you know only to kill those who follow you! The many very dear
relatives and friends you have killed are the ones, who, not believing
me because of you, I could now be enjoying! But you could not kill me
although you would have willingly done so, and in spite of you, I am
alive. And so I have come to that advanced age when I can enjoy my
eleven grandchildren, all very intelligent and kind in nature, gifted in
letters, well mannered, all full of life and in optimal form. But had I followed you I would not be enjoying them, nor my comfortable and beautiful residence – which I built – and its many secluded gardens that, to

---

63 Cornaro's judgment is common to notions held by Church, state, and society in
    Venice (and elsewhere) throughout history toward the "deserving" poor versus the
    "unworthy" or "idle" poor. Robert Jütte, for example, states that "Poverty as such was
    not degrading. However, as early as the fifteenth century the distinction between
    the deserving and undeserving poor became part of the discriminatory social policy
    towards beggars ... Whether or not they were regarded as victims of circumstances or
    were held responsible for their present miserable condition ... The pauper is often
    reduced to another stereotype, that of the sturdy beggar, unworthy of charity, on
    the one hand, and that of the cheerful, thankful, domestic and labouring poor on
    the other hand," *Poverty and Deviance in Early Modern Europe* (Cambridge: Cambridge
    University Press, 2001), p. 189. Cf. Ficino's comment, p. 29n46.

    For a brief time in the 1590s, the poor in Italy found a Robin Hood figure in the
    daring exploits of the brigand and mercenary Marco Sciarra of Abruzzo, who alleg-
    edly showed his respect to the renowned poet of *Gerusalemme liberate*, Torquato Tasso
    (1544–1595), during a robbery by allowing Tasso's carriage to proceed unmolested.
    Sciarra, who was eventually killed by order of Pope Clement VIII, "described himself
    as a 'scourge of God and envoy of God against usurers and the possessors of unpro-
    ductive wealth.'" Also see Piero Camporesi's investigation into the politic of bread
    and official and private policies toward the "*vero*" (true) poor and the undeserving
    poor, in *Il Pane selvaggio* (1980); English translation by David Gentilcore, *Bread of
    Dreams* (1989). On another context for Cornaro's comments, see above, note 58.

make perfect, took a very long time. But you kill whoever follows you, before their buildings and gardens can be finished, and yet I have already been enjoying mine for these many years, much to your confusion. But because you are a vice so pestilent that you foul and poison the entire world, and wanting with all my power to liberate the world of your part in it, I have resolved to work against you in this manner: my eleven grandchildren, after I have gone, will be the ones to make known the evil and corruption that you are – the mortal enemy of all men born.

To be sure, many of those who admire me, men of great intelligence, which they truly have and who have achieved a high standing in letters, as in other things, do not keep to that life; at least not until the age of fifty or sixty years, after they begin to feel the effects of some illness mentioned above. Because then they could easily decide [to adopt a sober life], since that illness, now old, is incurable. And I do not marvel at the young, because that age is governed by the senses, and their life is governed by those; but certainly once past fifty years, it is an age that in all things should be governed by reason, which makes known that to satisfy a person's tastes and appetites, is infirmity and death. And if the pleasure of tasting were to last a long time, it could be accepted, but no sooner has it begun then it is over, and the infirmities that come from it last a long time. But it is certain there is great happiness for the one living a sober life, for as soon as he has eaten he is certain that this food will keep him healthy, and that he could never become ill from it.

I had wanted to keep this addition to my Treatise to a few words, but for other reasons: because a lengthy read is seen by a few, while a short one is seen by many and I would like many to read it and so benefit those many.

(1561)

Letter Written by the Magnificent Alvise Cornaro to the Most Reverend Barbaro, Patriarch Elect of Aquileia[64]

Most Reverend Lordship,

Truly the intellect of man has something of the divine, and what a divine thing it was when it found the means through writing to converse with another far away. It was then completely divine for Nature to have the one so far away see the other through the eyes of thought, as I am seeing your Lordship, and in this manner to converse with you on agreeable things that benefit us a great deal. It is very true that it will be talk about a matter discussed at other times, but not at this my age of ninety-one years,[65] something I cannot overlook, because the more my years increase the more my prosperity increases, an effect that astonishes everyone. And I, knowing by which line of reasoning to proceed, am compelled to demonstrate it and let it be known that we can have earthly paradise after the age of eighty, which is [where] I am; but we cannot have it without the means of blessed Continence and the virtuous life of Sobriety much beloved by Our Great Lord, because they are enemies of the senses and friends of reason.

Now then, Lordship, by way of explanation, I will tell you that over these past days there have been many excellent Physicians around me – those who teach at the university, philosophers as much as doctors – very well informed on my age, the way I live, and my habits, knowing

---

64 Daniele Barbaro (1514–70), patron of the arts, illustrious exemplar of the Venetian Renaissance, deemed a worthy successor to Bembo, was a Venetian ambassador to London, nephew of Cardinal Francesco Pisani (with whom Cornaro had a clamorous falling out) and a participant at the Council of Trent in 1562.

65 In 1563 Cornaro is either seventy-nine or eighty-one years old.

how very happy and healthy I was; and that all my sensory capacities
were perfect, in addition to my memory, heart, intelligence, as well
as my voice and teeth. Moreover, they knew I was writing by hand for
eight hours a day on treatises beneficial to all mankind, and that I
spent many other hours walking and at other times singing – (such a
beautiful voice is mine, Lordship, that if you were to hear me singing
my prayers while accompanied by a harp, like David,[66] I assure you that
you would very much enjoy how melodiously I sing!). Further to what
the above physicians had to say, they again said that my writing so much
on matters intellectual and spiritual was certainly a wonderful thing (it
is, your Lordship, an incredible thing of pleasure and satisfaction that
I enjoy with these writings, but given that my writing is meant to be
beneficial, you yourself, Lordship, can understand how very great is my
pleasure). Finally, they said that I could not have been taken for an old
man because my actions were those of someone young and not those of
other old men, who, having reached eighty years, have all the actions of
the old. Besides, those defective with gout or their side or other ills, in
order to be free of them, are continually subjected to pills and bloodlet-
ting and medicines of other similar crazes, which are truly aggravating.
And even if there is someone free of infirmities, his sensory capacities
then suffer, whether it be his sight or hearing or one of the others such
as not being able to walk, or hands that tremble. And even if there was
someone free of such contraries, his memory is not perfect, nor his
heart or intellect, nor would his life be happy, satisfied, or as pleasurable as is mine. But one [blessing] – apart from the many others that
I did possess in the extreme – was puzzling, because it is completely
unnatural that I could keep myself alive these [past] fifty years despite
having this extreme contrary inside me, which is utterly fatal. But it is
something one cannot prepare against because it is a natural and occult property in my body placed there by Nature. So it is that every year
from the beginning of July until the end of August, during these two
months, I cannot drink wine, whether it is wine from some preferred
grape or wine from some preferred region; for during that time, wine,
in addition to being completely contrary to and the enemy of my taste,
is harmful to my stomach. And so having lost my milk – wine really being milk for the old[67] – and not having a way to drink, since waters that

---

66 "And so it was, whenever the spirit from God was upon Saul, that David would take a
   harp and play *it* with his hand. Then Saul would become refreshed and well, and the
   distressing spirit would depart from him," I Samuel 16:23, *NKJV*.
67 Proverbial (possibly Galenic): Vinum lac senum, "Wine is milk for the old."

have been altered and prepared cannot have the power of wine and do not benefit me,[68] thus, having nothing to drink and with my stomach unwell, I am unable to eat except for very little. And this eating little without any wine had reduced me by mid-August to a state of utmost fatal weakness. Capon broth did not help me nor any other remedy, so that as a result of my weakness I was close to death and not for any other ailment than out of sheer weakness; and they [physicians] concluded that if the new wine – which I always have readied at the beginning of September – were to be late, it would be the cause of my death. Nevertheless, they were more stupefied that this new wine, in a matter of two or three days, had the power to restore the prosperity that the old wine had taken from me; because in these past few days they had seen something that no one would have believed unless they had seen it for themselves. "It has been over many years now," —they said— "that various doctors among us have attended to him, and it has already been ten years since it was [first] thought he could not possibly live beyond one or two years at most with so mortal an illness as in these past years. And yet we see that this year you [*sic*] have been less weak." This, and the many other blessings found in me, led them to conclude that all my many blessings concentrated into one was a special blessing within me, granted to me at birth by Nature or the Heavens. And from a desire to prove good their conclusion (which is false, because it is not based on either a solid foundation or reasoning but on their own opinions) they were compelled to say beautiful and lofty things with supreme eloquence. To be sure, your Lordship, eloquence is most compelling in a man of high intelligence, [it is] sufficient to make even what is not [believable], nor can ever be, seem believable. Listening to them amused me and gave me great pleasure, because it really is very amusing to hear these discussions among those persons.[69]

Another pleasure I took complete satisfaction in at the time – considering that a long life of experience has the power to make someone who is not learned, learned, as this is the true foundation of the true sciences – was that in this way I knew their conclusion to be

---

68 A possible reference to water "altered" with additives such as wine, honey, salt, parsley, or vinegar, according to Roman or medieval treatments: See for example, Paolo Squatriti, *Water and Society in Early Medieval Italy AD 400–1000* (Cambridge: Cambridge University Press, 1998), p. 40. These "altered" waters are the likely precursors to *grappa,* and *aqua vitae* and "spirits" in general.

69 Cornaro was not enthralled with physicians of the time. See "Intro.," p. 10.

false; and so you see, Lordship, how men can fool themselves with their own opinions when they are not founded upon a real foundation. To dissuade them and to help them, I responded that their conclusion was false, as in fact I would have them see that the blessing in me is not special, but common, and that every man is able to enjoy it. Because I am but a mere man the same as everyone else, composed of the four elements and that, apart from my being and living, I have all five of my senses, my intelligence and reason. Every man is born with intelligence and reason, because Our Great Lord had willed that His man, whom He loves very much, would have more of these benefits and blessings than would animals – which have only their senses – so that man, with those benefits and blessings, might conserve his health for a long time. This blessing is thus a universal one conceded by God, and not by Nature or the Heavens. But when young, being more sensual than rational, a man followed his senses, and having now arrived at the age of forty or fifty years, he should know that he has then reached the midpoint of his life, by the advantage of his youth and his young stomach – natural advantages that had advanced his growth – but that he has now entered his decline toward death, by the disadvantage of old age; and that old age is contrary to youth, just as disorder is contrary to order. [He should further know] that it is necessary therefore to change his life in what he eats and drinks, in that a long and a healthy life depends upon it; and that, with the first half of his life having been a sensual one without order, the second half must be one of reason, with order. Because without order nothing can be conserved, the life of man even less than any other thing, as it is a known fact that disorder is harmful and order is beneficial. And in Nature, it is not possible that someone wanting to satisfy his taste and his appetites does not [in this way] cause disorder; and as for me, so as not to cause disorder, having reached a mature age, I have taken up the life of order and sobriety.

The truth is, I had difficulty removing myself from a life of non-sobriety, and to do it, I first prayed to God that He grant me His virtue of restraint [*continenza*], knowing that my prayer would be heard. Then – knowing this – when a man wishes to undertake a good effort, which he knows he can do though with difficulty, he can still facilitate it through stubborn resolve in wanting to do it, and he does it; and so it was I became resolute. What is more, I undertook to remove myself little by little from a disordered life, and so little by little placed myself into an ordered one. And in this way I adopted the sober life, so later it did not bother me, even though I was compelled in that life to adhere most strictly to the quality and quantity of my foods and wine, having as

I do the poorest of complexions. But those with a good [[complexion]] can eat many other kinds and qualities of food, and in greater quantity, and likewise drink wine; so that although his life is a sober one it will not therefore be a restricted life as is mine, but more open.[70]

Having heard my reasoning and having seen the fundamentals, everyone concluded that I had said all there was to say. But one, the youngest, said he would concede that this blessing was universal but that I, at least, had had this special blessing of being easily able to remove myself from one life and to put myself into another; something that in his experience he found possible to do, but for him it was with the greatest of difficulty whereas for me it had been easy. I told him that being a man like himself it was still difficult for me, but that it is not an honest thing for a man to leave a beautiful undertaking – one which he is capable of doing – and to abandon it because of its difficulty, for the more difficult it is the more honour he attains. And he does what to God is more blessed, because the Will [of God] – since He has established life as being one hundred years for man[71] – is for all men to arrive at that age, knowing that once man passes his eightieth year he is free of all the bitter fruit of the senses, and filled with those of sacred reason, so that vices and sins are compelled to leave him. Therefore, this God desires that man live a long life, and He has ordained that the one to live to his natural end, as indicated above, may finish his life free of illness and out of resolution. This is a natural end, and the exiting of a mortal life to enter one immortal, as will happen to me when I am certain I will die singing my prayers.[72] Nor does the dreadful thought of death disturb me now – even if I know very well that a long life brings me closer to it – thinking about how I was born to die, and that many have died at a younger age than

---

70 "There is a risk that the reader of the *Vita sobria*," Milani advises, "fascinated and intrigued by the details of this most strange diet as described – may forget that Cornaro only speaks of this as an example, rather, a point of reference for anyone who wishes to undertake the path of sobriety, but he was always careful to advise that what may have been good for him cannot work for everyone and that each person, being the ideal physician for [oneself], can find a suitable and effective diet": see "Intro.," p. 25.

71 Different Bible passages yield a different life expectancy for man, for example, in Psalms 90:10, it is seventy or eighty years, in Genesis 6:2–4, it is 120 years.

72 Cornaro had written of singing in his eulogy, yet his grandson Giacomo Alvise, in a letter dated "the end of April 1566," writes that although his grandfather was rational, his tongue was quite swollen, which would suggest he was unable to sing (*Sober* ..., p. 181). Also see M.A. Graziani's account of Cornaro's death, "Intro," p. 43n73. On the spiritual significance of song, see "Eulogy," p. 132n2.

mine. Nor does the other thought – companion to the one above – trouble me, which is fear of the pains that we suffer for our sins after death; because I am a good Christian, and I must believe I will be free of them by the power of the most Sacred Blood of Christ, Who wished it shed in order to free us, His faithful Christians, from those pains. O what a beautiful life is mine! O what a happy ending will be mine!

After I had finished saying all of this, the young man said nothing in reply except that he was determined to take up the sober life and further prolong his life as I had done, and that he would do another very important thing since he was rather troubled over growing older – he now wanted to grow old little by little and so enjoy his enjoyable old age.

My great desire to speak with you, most Reverend Lordship, has made me go on at length and makes me speak further, but only briefly. There are those who are very sensual, Lordship, who say I have wasted my time and labour on writing my Treatise on the Sober Life, and so it will lay there because it is impossible to do, and the treatise will have been in vain, as was Plato's *Republic*. [Plato,] who toiled away writing something that could not be carried out, and similarly institute a Republic that neither he nor others have ever, nor will ever, institute; and so his treatise was in vain, as will be mine. I marvel a great deal at them, since they can also read in my treatise that I maintained a sober life for many years before writing about it, and I would not have written it had I not seen beforehand that it was a life one can lead, and how greatly it benefitted me, and that it was a virtuous life. And with my being indebted to it, I was compelled to write about it so that it may be known for what it is. I know that after reading my treatise many have taken up that life and as we know many in the past have maintained it, so that the opposition that befell that of the *Republic* will not befall my *Vita sobria*.

*[[And further to those sensual men, the enemies of reason and friends of sensuality, taste and appetite, in order to excuse and defend their vices – which truly are the ones that kill men before their time, for it is not possible that in Nature those wishing to indulge their senses, their tastes, and their appetites, are not by these means preparing for their infirmity and death, as we see every day in those who are sensual – but, as was said, in order to remove that infamy from the senses, they

---

* Paragraph between double brackets was omitted by Cornaro's grandson, Giacomo Alvise. See "Intro.," p. 32.

say that when a young man dies, he died because he arrived at the end
of his life, ended by God. And in their defence they plead the Holy
Scripture, where it says God had affixed an end to the life of man,
which cannot be exceeded; it is true that He did affix one, and that
it cannot be exceeded, but it is not what they understand it to mean
whenever someone dies. Nor does it say so in the Holy Scripture, nor
does it mean that [particular] ending of life but a general ending –
which is general to all men – and the actual true ending of life ended
by God, which is that a man can live up to the age of one hundred
years; and it is this end to life that cannot be exceeded, either by Continence or a sober life. And if it was the [end] that they say, which is one
whereby a man dies before his time, it would then be by a Partial and
Unjust God depriving a person of life before his time, and not allowing
him to enjoy the most perfect age, which is once he has passed eighty
years. Because this is an age full of reason, experience, knowledge,
goodness and charity, free of sin and therefore much beloved by God.
We must believe that He would want every man to enjoy that age, and
it is to this outcome that He gave to man reason and intellect that with
these he could arrive at that age – but man does not wish to give up
his sensuality nor taste nor appetites and will therefore die before his
time.]]*

(1563)

---

* End of the omitted paragraph.

A Loving Exhortation by the Magnificent Messer Alvise Cornaro

in which by true reasoning he persuades every person to lead an Ordered and Sober Life relevant to reaching old age when Man may enjoy all the Blessings and benefits that God in His Goodness consents to grant Mortals.

THE TRUE WAY TO LIVE A LONGER LIFE AND THE BLESSINGS AND BENEFITS TO BE ENJOYED IN OLD AGE

Not to neglect the obligation to which every living being is held, and so as not to lose altogether the great pleasure I find in being helpful, I wanted to write this and let those who do not know – not practising [a sober life] – all that is known and understood by the ones who practise what I do. And because, to some, certain things seemed impossible and difficult to believe though nonetheless true – being and seeing these things for themselves in actuality – I will not be remiss in writing them down for the benefit of everyone. And on this, I say, having reached (by God's Grace) the age of ninety-five years[73] and finding myself healthy, prosperous, happy and content, I continue to give praise to His Divine Majesty for the many blessings given me, as I see that typically among all other older men, once they reach seventy years, they are in poor health, prospering less, melancholic and discontent. Constantly thinking about death and believing day after day that they are about to die, it will therefore be almost impossible to rid their minds of that thought. The thought does not disturb me at all because I cannot think about such a thing in any way, as I will later demonstrate more clearly; moreover, I will plainly demonstrate the confidence I have for living to the age of one hundred years. But, to better organize my writing, I will begin with the birth of a man, and so discussing, arrive at his death.

---

73 In 1565 Cornaro is either eighty-one or eighty-three years old.

I would say, therefore, that some are born so scarcely alive they live only a few days or months or years, and it is not well understood if the cause of so short a life comes from a defect of the father or of the mother in conceiving him, or the revolutions of the Heavens, or a defect of Nature, which still comes from those Heavens, and so I can never believe that, being the Mother of everyone, she could be partial about her children. Therefore, not being able to know the cause is to rely by necessity on what everyday can be seen as fact. Others are born quite lively and healthy, but with a poor and weak complexion, and some among these live to the age of ten, some to twenty, others to thirty or forty years, but not one reaches an old age.[74] Others are born with a perfect complexion and do reach old age, but for the most part they are old persons poorly conditioned (as I indicated above); and for this poor condition and indisposition they themselves are the cause. It is because they rely too greatly, without reason, on their perfect complexion, and do not wish to change at all the way they live from the time they were young to when they are old, as if they still possessed the same vigour as before. They expect to live their old age in the same disordered way they did all throughout their youth, never thinking about growing old, much less that their complexion could lose its vigour. And they think even less so about their stomach having lost its natural heat, which is why they need to give more consideration to the quality of their food and wine, and to reduce their large quantity. Yet, contrarily, they try to increase it, saying that as man loses his prosperity due to old age, it must be conserved with more quantities of food, since eating is what conserves man in life. So it is they go far in fooling themselves because just as man is going to lose heat as he ages, so it is his task to reduce his food and drink, since Nature is content with little in order to conserve the old. And though the old should in all good reason believe this, instead they do not and continue to follow their usual disordered life; yet, had they stopped at that time and had they begun a life of order and sobriety, they would have grown older, as I have done, being well conditioned. And they, having been born by the Grace of the Great Lord with such a good and perfect complexion, would live to one hundred and twenty years, just as others have

---

74 In 1564 his two grandsons, Fantino and Ferigo, died while very young at twenty-four and twenty-three years of age, respectively. His brother Giacomo had died in 1541, close friends Ruzzante in 1542 and Falconetti in 1535. With their deaths, Cornaro was to adjust his position on a sober life having the power to conserve everyone, see "Intro.," pp. 19–20.

done who maintained a sober life – which we hear about everywhere – by reason of having been born with this perfect complexion. Had I too been born with one, I certainly would have no doubt about reaching that age, but because I was born with a poor one, I doubt I will live beyond one hundred years, which is the same for others similarly born with a poor one. For if they were to follow an ordered life as I have done, they would then reach one hundred years or more in good health, as will I. This certainty of living for many years seems to me a beautiful thing and is to be greatly respected, since we know of no one who can be sure of living for even one hour except for those who maintain a sober life, whose foundation and surety for living is based upon sound and true natural reasons, which cannot be denied. Because in Nature it is not possible that someone who keeps an ordered and sober life could ever become ill, or die an unnatural death before his time; seeing that, when it is his time he must necessarily die, but not to die before his time. And it is because this sober life has the virtue of removing all the causes that cause illness, and illness cannot occur without a cause, and with that cause removed the illness is removed and with the illness removed so too is an unnatural death. There is no doubt that an ordered and sober life, which has the virtue and power to remove those causes that cause illness, is what operates the humours; and the humours keep a man healthy or ill, alive or dead. And since there are good humours and bad, the sober life operates so that the bad, being bad, are changed into good and perfect ones. The sober life thus has this natural virtue of operating on the humours, which, perforce, unite, adapt and bind together in such a way they can no longer be separated, activated, or altered into becoming those things that give rise to cruel fever and an ultimately death.

It is very true and cannot be denied that even before being made good, it is yet possible that time, the consumer of all things, could consume and even resolve those humours; and that once consumed it is better for man to die a natural death without ailments. It will happen to me that I die at my time, when these humours will have been consumed, which at present they have not been, rather, they are good. Nor could it be otherwise, since I am so healthy, happy, and content, and have a good appetite and sleep peacefully; moreover, my sensory capacities are all healthy and perfect. My intellect is as sharp and clear as ever, my judgment sound, my memory unwavering, my heart big, and my voice, which before tended to be lower, is stronger and has become melodious, and I am now obliged to sing my morning and evening prayers in a loud voice, whereas once I spoke them in a subdued and low one. And these are all real and certain indications and signs that my humours are good and cannot be consumed, except over time, as all those who practise as I do will find.

O what a glorious life will be mine! A life full of all the contentment to be enjoyed on earth, and it is also (as it truly is) free of animal sensuality, which is driven out by virtue of a long life. Because where reason is, sensuality has no place, nor its bitter fruits, which are the passions, perturbations, and bad thoughts. Nor is there a place in me for the thought of death, there being nothing of the sensual in me; nor can the death of my grandsons or other relatives or friends upset me if not as a first impulse,[75] but it is soon gone; and the losses of my business dealings upset me even less (as many have seen, to their great admiration). But this can only happen to someone who grows old by means of a sober life, not by a strong complexion, and who will also happily enjoy his life as I do in continuous good times [*sollazzo*] and pleasure.

Who would not enjoy his life, not having any adversity at such an old age? And since others who are younger do have them – of which, as we know, they have an infinite number – I will now more clearly demonstrate that they do not have any of my pastimes. The first of these is to help your beloved homeland, for what a glorious pastime this is and one I immensely enjoy, because in demonstrating the way to safeguard her most important lagoon and port – to ensure that it not deteriorate before thousands of years have passed – Venice will conserve her marvellous and splendid name of the Virgin City, which she is, as there is no other like her in the world; furthermore, it will enhance her great and lofty title of Queen of the Sea, and I take great pleasure in this, as there is nothing I would not provide for her. Another pastime I enjoy is in demonstrating to this Virgin and Queen, the means to render her bountiful in foodstuffs by converting her unutilized fields into fields of great utility – be they marshlands or dry lands – yielding great profit over the cost. And I enjoy this other pastime, which is unopposed, in which I demonstrate to Venice the way to become more powerful though already very powerful and unconquerable, more beautiful though already very beautiful, wealthier though already very wealthy, and to improve her air

---

75 On *sensual,* see above, note 19, and see "Terminology": *Coitus, Sensual.* Galen condemns "psychic pain" as an emotion, and "congratulates himself for his conquest of it," Susan Mattern, *Galen and the Rhetoric of Healing* (Baltimore: Johns Hopkins University Press, 2008), p. 134.

though already perfect. These are the three pastimes, all in the name of helping, which I enjoy with immense satisfaction. And who could find anything contrary in these when none exist?

I take pleasure as well in this other, for which – having lost a considerable amount of revenue, leaving my grandchildren deprived owing to this misfortune – by my intellect alone, which does not sleep, and not by physical exertion – if not for a little of the mind [*mente*] – I have found a true and infallible way to restore that damage [of lost revenue] twofold, by means of proper and worthy agriculture.

Another pastime I still enjoy is my Treatise I wrote to help others, on the Sober Life, and which I see does help, as some confirm to me personally that it benefits them a great deal – which in fact can be seen – and others in their letters say that their life, after God, relies upon me.

There is still one more pastime I enjoy, which is the writing I do by my own hand and so I write a great deal in order to be helpful, be it on architecture,[76] or agriculture. Another thing I enjoy is conversing with men of great and high intelligence, from whom even at this age I can still learn. What delight it is, that at this age we do not tire of learning something great, however lofty and difficult it may be.

I would like to add – though to some it seems impossible and could never be – that at this age I suddenly enjoy two lives: the one terrestrial through effect, and the second celestial through thought. The latter has the virtue to be enjoyed, when founded on a thing that is to be enjoyed, as I am certain that I will enjoy it out of the infinite Goodness and Mercy of Our Great Lord. So it is I enjoy this earthly one, thanks to an ordered and sober life, most grateful to her Majesty [Nature] as she is full of virtue and the enemy of vice. And I enjoy (by the Grace of this Great Lord) the celestial – which He ensures I enjoy by means of my thought, which has taken away my ability to think of anything else – as what I believe and affirm to be more than certain. And I believe that our dying is not dying but a transition our soul makes from this earthly life to the one celestial, immortal, and infinitely perfect; and it could not be otherwise. This lofty thought is raised so high that it can no longer descend to the common and mundane – that of the dying of this body – but only to living a life celestial and divine, thus I have come to enjoy two lives. Nor can its ending – and the great enjoyment I have in this life now – bring

---

76 On Cornaro's architectural "constructions," see for example, Manfredo Tafuri, *Venezia e il Rinascimento* (Torino: Giuli Einaudi, 1985); *Venice and the Renaissance*, trans. Jessica Levine (Cambridge, MA: MIT Press, 1995).

me any harm, but rather such great infinite joy, for its ending marks the beginning of another glorious life, celestial and immortal.

And who could be troubled by so great a good, so great a happiness, and so great a grace as will be mine? It is something every other man would have who follows the life I have led, which anyone can follow, as I am no more than a man, not a saint but a servant of God, to Whom that life of order is most pleasing. And because many men take up a holy and beautiful and spiritual and contemplative life filled with prayer, if they were only to give themselves completely to an ordered and sober life, how much more grateful they would be to our Supreme Lord! They would also make the world beautiful and so be held on earth as true Holy fathers, as once were held to be the ancients, who observed the sober life along with the spiritual.[77] Similarly, living to the age of one hundred-twenty years by virtue of God, they would also perform countless miracles, as the ancients did; furthermore, they would always be healthy, content, and happy, where, for the most part, now they are unhealthy, melancholic, and discontent. And since some who believe that these things were given to them for the good of their health by our Great Lord and thus are able, in this life, to pay penitence for their errors, in my judgment they are fooling themselves; as I cannot believe the Lord would ever have His man, whom He loves a great deal, live being ill and melancholic and discontent, but rather, healthy and happy and content. Because it was also in this way that the Holy Fathers lived, and they were then always better servants to His Almighty, performing the many beautiful miracles we read about.

How beautiful and enjoyable a world it would be now, as it was then, and even more beautiful, if – given the many Religions and Monasteries now that did not exist at that time – had a sober life been maintained, we would be seeing such a wealth of venerable old men that it would be a wonder. Nor because of this would an ordered life be absent among religions, rather it would proliferate, because to all religions it is conceded, in order to live, the eating of bread and the drinking of wine, and at times some eggs as well and at other times some meat. In addition to which there are legume soups, salads, fruits, and egg tarts; foods that are often harmful, by which some have lost their lives. But because they

---

77 Followers of the eremitic Christian tradition, or Hermits, elect for a solitary life
   (Desert Theology of the Old Testament) in spiritual devotion and prayer to God, and
   hence benefit their fellow man during their encounters with them.

are [foods] conceded to them by their Orders, they make use of them, perhaps thinking that omitting them would be in error, which it is not. Rather, they would do very well if once past the age of thirty years they were to omit those and begin to live on bread in wine, a *panatella* of bread, and eggs with bread; this is the true life for conserving a man of poor complexion. And it is a life more open than the one followed in the desert among the ancient Holy Fathers, who ate only wild fruit and herb roots and drank plain water, and yet they lived as I have said for a long time being healthy, happy, and content. So too will those of our own times, and together they will find the way to Heaven more easily, which always remains open to every faithful Christian. So it was that Christ Our Redeemer left [Heaven] when He descended from above, coming to earth to shed His precious blood and free us from tyrannical servitude to the Devil, and all this He did out of His infinite Goodness.

And so to conclude my line of reasoning, I say that, with an advanced age being (as it truly is) full and overflowing with many blessings and benefits – myself, besides, being one of those to enjoy them – I cannot be remiss (not wanting to be lacking in charity) in bearing witness and in completely assuring each person that there is much more I enjoy than what I have written here. And that the reason for my writing is nothing if not for the purpose – seeing the great good that comes from this long life – of having every person observe this great and commendable life of order and sobriety. To this end I will continue crying out – *Live! Live!* – *that you may better serve the Lord.*

(1565)

Eulogy for Alvise Cornaro[1]

O Great and Eternal God on High, Our Lord Jesus Christ, to You I turn my eyes, my mind, and my heart that You may grant me the grace to say all that I should, nor do I ask this of you Phoebus or of you Muses, as [the Lord] is high above you. Thus, it is to You Lord the First Cause that I pray,* that granting me [grace] might please You, for without it I could not nor would I know how to speak of the many virtues of this man so rare, filled with continence, charity, goodness, beautiful manners, but who, above all else, was highly intelligent: virtues that those of you who came to hear me speak can attest. And since he was a man of high intelligence and I who speak of him of but a low one, for this reason Lord, raise me and give me the grace, style, and eloquence that I may properly speak of this man who was more than a father. For out of one who came from nothing, he has made a man, helping me learn to read, something that owing to my misfortune I did not know how to do. And later, my being ill at the age of ten – when doctors and their many medicines could never free me of my malady – I was freed of it when he demonstrated to me the one true and natural medicine, which is Continence, the mother of a Sober Life.

Having therefore so great a debt to this man, it is necessary to have from You, Great Lord, a way to speak of him, and even more so since he

---

1 Cornaro had allegedly written his own eulogy, but as Milani points out, it should not be surprising since it was not unheard of at the time to write one's own epigraph (e.g., S. Speroni), see "Intro.," p. 41. Orazio Lovato, a young protégé of Cornaro, was identified by Paolo Sambin as the one who read the eulogy at Cornaro's funeral, not his grandson Giacomo Alvise, see "Intro.," p. 41.

* See "Terminology," *Cause.*

died in my arms singing Bembo's beautiful devotional prayer, and as the prayer ended, so too his life ended.[2] At his ending there were many who had come to contemplate and to view him, and they saw that he ended without pain.

O blessed soul – by the Grace of God how you rose up to Heaven on your good wings[3] to live a better life, the one eternal, and you left us to much weeping and tears that fill me once again. Free me of them Lord, I pray You, that my grief does not take away from what I must say, as I know Your Lord wishes me to speak on the life and customs of one who was so much Yours. Luigi Cornaro, born in Venice – a relative fourth removed from Marco Cornaro, the Doge[4] – who should have been named Cornelio because that was his true family name, as confirmed by Roman as well as Venetian histories and archives, because the house of Cornaro descended from the Sipioni Cornelii who came to Venice to settle, having been driven away by warring factions [in Morea]; and just as changes to language occasionally occur, their surname changed from Cornelio to Cornaro. So it was the very wealthy son of the said Doge – given the great friendship between the despots of Morea (part of Greece)[5] and himself – by using a portion of his wealth, acquired a piece of their territory which was then held by his family for eighty-five years. Not having any of their noble descendants oversee their Venetian nobility, and

---

2 This was not to be. See "Intro.," p. 65 and see *Sober ...*, p. 181. Cornaro's insistence on the power of his voice may have to do with Ficino (after Plato) who states that "song is nothing else but another spirit." With this, according to Giuseppe Mazzotta, Ficino "articulates his theory of the superiority of the sense of hearing over the other senses. Words, songs and sounds are privileged vehicles for reaching the rational faculty of the soul. Thus along with his father Phoebus, Orpheus is the figure of the poet who performs miracles with the enchantment of his song," *Cosmospoeisis: The Renaissance Experiment* (2001), p. 13.

3 A possible reference to the wings of an angel, or the soul: "The soul is thought of as the perfected *imago* escaping from the *pupa*, just as the word *Psuchē* or Psyche meant in Greek the moth or butterfly." *Marcus Aurelius: Meditations*, trans. A.S.L. Farquharson, intro. D.A. Rees (New York: Random House, 1992), p. 225.

4 If true, then Marco Cornaro (1286?–1368), the Doge of Venice from 1365–1368, would have been Cornaro's great-great-great-great-grandfather. See "Intro.," p. 46n78. Rigo (Enrico), the disreputable son of the Doge, had been charged with murder and banished from Venice.

5 Morea (or Peloponnesos), from the mid-1300s to 1460, was part of the Eastern Roman (Byzantine) Empire. Thomas and Demetrios II, the brothers of the region's last ruling Roman emperor, Constantine XI Palaiologos, were the joint despots of the Morea until driven out by the Ottomans in 1460.

being abroad, they did not observe the regulatory laws by which, when a noble is born he is to be notarized in the public records; and for not having themselves notarized, their nobility was lost. It was thus in this way it was lost to them. And the Great Turk[6] – with whom the aforementioned despots exchanged only much love – changed his love into hate and displeasure and resolved to take the territory from them; and since the land belonging to the Cornaro was part of that territory, he wanted it back. They [Cornaro] were then forced to return to Venice, albeit with greater means of money, silver, and goods not being less than the amount his relatives had brought to that country.

Into this branch of the family Luigi was born, with a fine intellect and a kind nature, which could be seen by the age of ten; he applied himself to the study of letters and by the age of fifteen was quite well read. He was very congenial, witty, and as has been said, a good companion, for which he was well liked by other young people his age. Understanding this, he decided to organize a [theatre] group, as is the tradition in Venice, called the *Compagnia di Calza*,[7] which was most beautiful and enjoyable. It was the first to perform comic plays – previously not the custom in Venice – which were performed in a charming way by company members; and the intermissions were similarly done with ideal music that was most beautiful and enjoyable, because among their group were four of the most beautiful voices. It was for this company that he composed songs, lyrics and comedies, which were full of genuine laughter, and for four years the city was kept wonderfully entertained and charmed.

By the age of twenty-two he decided to pursue his studies here in Padua – studying law to defend causes – where he remained for two years, learning a great deal. But considering that Venetian laws were

---

6 The "Great Turk" likely refers to Fatih Sultan Mehmet II (1432–1481) "the Conqueror," who captured Constantinople in 1453.

7 *Compagnia della Calza*, [stocking group or "gang"] was the name of a number of theatrical companies in the Veneto (1450s–1560s), which entertained during *Carnevale*, fêtes, or visits by dignitaries. They were "festive clubs of young nobles known for their hedonism and for pushing the limits of their elders' tolerance." Given their anti-authoritarian posture, members were to "keep secret the affairs of the company," Edward Muir, *The Culture Wars* …, (Cambridge, MA: Harvard University Press, 2007), pp. 126–7. Each company had its own distinguishing name, colour and embroidered stocking (*calza*) worn by its noble class (only) members. Though lacking a noble title, Cornaro was an associate and patron of the company of the white-stocking *Zardinieri* or *Giardinieri* [Gardeners] gang. See "Intro.," pp. 46–7, and p. 46n80.

  Writings on the Sober Life

different from the ones he was studying, and that in Venice defending
causes was conducted in another manner, he returned to Venice at the
age of twenty-four. He studied Venetian statutes and learned the practice, then he put himself to work defending causes, for which he did
very well, although it was not work he enjoyed. And with his good fortune wanting him to do something worthy of his intellect, finding himself in possession of two hundred fields of marshlands – acquired from
relatives[8] – which, because of their continuous running water, were full
of reeds, he undertook to see if the fields could be cleared of that water
and so be cultivated. His own reasoning on the matter (to which, we
later learned, he had given a great deal of thought) found that the fields
could be dried, but that it would be expensive. To proceed with this, he
sold and used what little means he had as collateral in order to drain the
fields and to purchase other similar lands with marshes; and he bought
another five hundred that in less than two years had all been farmed.
The air then improved over that habitation and over that location, where
once the air had been so poor that babies newly born could not be saved;
and with the waters gone, the foul air ceased and good air returned,
where once there were forty souls there are now two thousand. He
made excellent income for his expertise, and for the church, a church
once rather ugly he later made beautiful. So one could say that in that
place he brought to God a temple, an altar, and the souls to adore Him;
and he always took care of those souls with the two priests of letters and
music. He then made himself a comfortable and proper rural villa built
according to architectural principles – so beautiful, so soundly built, and
so comfortable, it is unique to those surroundings – which he wanted to
face with stone and so safeguard it against fire, war, and anything else.
He had a number of dwellings built for the farmers, and a bridge made
to cross the Brenta River, which flowed through the middle of that complex; work done not just by one man but as a communal effort. And in
that villa he established a wonderful tradition, whereby, when one was
or is offended by another, peace is made right away; and so accordingly,

---

8 From his father Antonio – who was from the family of the Corner/Cornaro – Cornaro,
  along with his mother, inherited the Palazzo San Bartolamio where he had been born.
  It is thought to have been sold by Cornaro in the 1540s to raise money and so avoid
  going to prison for his debts. His maternal uncle, Giacomo Angelieri (d.1511?), a
  wealthy and powerful prior of the Collegio Pratense of Padua, bequeathed him various
  holdings, including the marshlands in Codevigo, with which Cornaro alleged he had
  generated his wealth. Also see "Intro.," pp. 46–9.

it is the villa of peace there, since the others are all full of discord and arms. He also introduced and taught residents the correct method for farming, which they had not known, and which later brought him great profit.

He built one of the finest gardens in the Este Hills, filled with various delicate fruits and the perfect grapes for making perfect wines; here in Padua, he then built the house we see, a kind not found in any other city. And being set in the most beautiful part he has surrounded it with six beautiful gardens of various forms – each adorned with different ornamentals – throughout which a wide and flowing river wends. In this house he built rooms that in winter remain warm without stoves or fireplaces, and in summer remain cool without ventilation or humidity. Having these beautiful and comfortable rooms, he lodged all the distinguished noblemen passing through this city, welcoming them into his spacious greenhouse with graciousness and unassuming courtesy. After having built such a beautiful residence, he decided on living in this city; and as soon as he heard of someone with a fine intellect, but who, owing to poverty, was unable to demonstrate it – whether in letters, poetry, music, painting, architecture, or sculpture – he would take that person under his care and provide him with the encouragement and means for him to express it.

In his youth he took great pleasure in hunting large animals such as goat, boar, and deer, and because none were found here in this town but in the area of Loreo – which is divided by a branch of the Po River – a lodge convenient for hunting was built above it. And every year for many years he went to hunt there, catching a number of those animals, which at times he would give away when in Venice, and other times when in Padua, he would send to nobles. At the end of hunting season, he organized a comedy to be performed in his theatre, built in imitation of ancient ones, for which he had the stage made out of durable stone, and in another section where the public stood he had benches placed that could later be removed. All of the comedies were successful, because staying in his home under his care were the many very talented male performers, such as the famous Ruzzante.[9]

---

9 Angelo Beolco (1502?–1542), known as Ruzzante (or Ruzante), the name of a comedic character he performed theatrically – and a sexual play on the verb *ruzzare*, to cavort – was the natural son of a Paduan academic-physician. Descended from Milanese nobility, the actor, playwright, musician, and member of the "Compagnia della Calza," also acted as an estate administrator for Cornaro. Called to the Este Court in Ferrara by Messisbugo

Through the disorders he had acquired from hunting and from other things, such as suffering the cold, heat, fatigue, and so on, not knowing what continence was nor a sober life, he fell ill at the age of thirty-five and remained so for five years, and neither the doctors' medicines nor bath cures could ever free him of this illness. After withdrawing from his treatment and case – no longer knowing which method could cure him – the doctors concluded they were unable to cure him for two reasons: first, because his was the result of a poor and a very sensual complexion; and second, because he had suffered endless disorders. Seeing that his doctors had abandoned him, he decided on medicating himself with a natural medicine, that of the [sober] diet, the daughter of great Continence, and he did not die; so that in a few months he was free of his illness. He got married and had a daughter, an only child,[10] and through her he wished to regain use of a noble title for his descendants; as he wanted her to marry the person within her lineage, a Cornaro progeny, among

---

(see *"Sober ...,"* p. 77n13), he had occasion to work with the great poet Ludovico Ariosto. Ruzzante's works were posthumously published, working in *pavano* – the literary parodic language that commingles the Paduan countryside dialect with other languages – he "employed peasant characters to satirize and sometimes bitterly criticize the pretension of the upper classes, and under the protection of his young patrons he pushed the limits of toleration," (E. Muir, *Culture Wars ...*, p. 127). After offending French dignitaries, in 1511, Beolco "never appeared on the Venetian stage again" (ibid.). "The theatrical career of Ruzante in Venice ended when, during an official party, he played a politically incorrect staging of a running decapitated rooster on the white linen of the table in front of the French Ambassador to the *Serenissima*. (In Italian, rooster and Gaul are identical words: *gallo*.)" Marco Frascari, "*Honestamente Bella*, Alvise Cornaro's Temperate View of Lady Architecture and Her Maids, Phronesis and Sophrosine" (http://www.arch.mcgill.ca/theory/conference/papers/Frascari_Cornaro.pdf), p. 19. 6 May 2013.

    Ruzzante and artist-architect Giovanni Maria Falconetto (1468–1535), along with family members and other noteworthy persons (Musso), all lived in the guest quarters of Cornaro's residence. Cornaro's Loggia, and Villa Cornaro, were in fact designed with Falconetto. Also see Richard Andrews, *Scripts and Scenarios* (1993), Emilio Lovarini, *Studi sul Ruzante e la letteratura pavana* (1965). The Italian comedic playwright Dario Fo, on the occasion of receiving his Nobel Prize for Literature in 1997, publicly acknowledged the influence of Ruzzante's comedic greatness. A brilliant playwright, Ruzzante predates Shakespeare.

10 Cornaro is said to have fathered two daughters, Chiara, with his wife Veronica Agugia da Spilimbergo, and later, Cornelia, with Petrinella da Armer di Candia, a vocalist of renown working with his theatre group – who had supposedly been Cornaro's lover for several years. See "Intro.," p. 51, p. 66, and p. 67n112. Cf. Paolo Sambin, *Per le biografie ...*, p. 128, where he holds that another Cornelia was his daughter.

the most handsome and brightest minds then in his homeland.[11] And though there were various high placed persons, in addition to the one cited, who were interested in her from various houses and other cities in Italy, he wished her to marry as chosen; and as a consequence, he gained numerous beautiful fine descendants. He therefore made five remarkable achievements: the first, as a landowner of commendable means; second, so rare and beautiful a house; third, his health; fourth, the use of his Venetian nobility, which cannot be purchased with money; fifth, his many remarkable descendants who will be his everlasting progeny.

Seeing the number of his grandchildren increase, he decided to increase his property and acquired two thousand fields of marshes for draining, one quarter of which had been drained within two years. And all would have been drained if envy had not led to a problem, for it was argued that the drainage was damaging the lagoon, which, however, was untrue; and the groups – which had brought that lawsuit and another, no less important, against him – had concluded that these [lawsuits] would show that if things had turned out happily for him, it was the result of his being fortunate but not of his intelligence. With two lawsuits having been served against him, he was not saddened but gladdened, saying God had sent them to him so that his constancy and good heart might be recognized once again, and so that he might willingly defend himself. And he won them, to his great advantage and honour;* and he ended up learning which methods were available to prevent the deterioration of the lagoon. Having witnessed these victories, everyone was forced to see that his business was not the result of luck but of his brilliant intellect; as truly this was so. And having learned to be an expert on the lagoon – since his homeland was suffering with the lagoon's deterioration – he advised them on the way to solve the problem; which he did solve, even though it would cause him harm, as we have seen and as came to be known. He then found a way for the area around Padua to be cleared of water, given that a quarter of his own land had remained with swamps and was not used. Now we can actually see how

---

11 Giovanni Alvise Cornaro Piscopia (1514–1559), the well regarded young, wealthy, and noble Venetian (descendant of the Cyprus Cornaro), married Cornaro's daughter Chiara with whom he had eleven children. Never particularly robust, he died while still a young man in his forties, after which Bishop Cornelio Musso wrote to Chiara saying that Giovanni was "more worthy of Heaven than earth," *Scritti ...*, p. 241.

* It is not known if he did win these lawsuits. See "Intro.," pp. 57–9.

these beautiful mountains – once surrounded by marshlands because of the water – after advising them on the way to drain them, are now cleared of water and made very beautiful; and how the countless owners of those places and other places like it have become wealthy. And so it can be seen that, from those parts of this territory, he removed the foul air and made it good and the town beautiful, and brought income to the land owners; things which have something of the divine.

To increase his earnings a third time for his large number of grand-children, he decided to sell his fields in Codevico [*sic*]. He found some-one who paid sixty ducats per field – and since he could buy a marshland for six ducats, which he knew could be drained at a cost of four ducats a field and then sell one field for sixty ducats – from that one tract of land he gained five or more usable lands, for which he earned a tremendous profit. However, his wife and daughter, in consideration of his eighty years and doubting that after draining the marshlands he would survive with his life, his being most dear to them, they pleaded with him not to make that sale or that purchase. And in order not to displease them, he complied, but now we know that had he done what he wanted, he would have acquired tremendous wealth.[12]

Truly, this was a man of high intelligence and impeccable judgment and one who was not presumptuous. He was sought by many noblemen who had wanted to make him a count, a doctor, or a knight; but he never wanted this. Nor did he ever want to eat from silver, nor dress in a showy manner, nor did he want many servants but only a few good ones, whom he paid well. And after they had been in his service for one year or more, he arranged their marriages with gifts or else found another way for them to live as free persons. He never wanted a large number of horses nor the expensive ones, but the modestly priced ones that were well suited as workhorses; he was the first to adopt a horse and carriage, finding it very convenient and very quick. For he was a man quick of action and whatever he had to do in a day he did not let slide into the next. He was very much an enemy of idleness, card playing, or games of dice. He spent his time studying and writing and thus wrote many trea-tises, all of which were helpful: the first on the sober life, the second on water conservation of his homeland and the reduction of marshlands, the third on architecture, the fourth on agriculture, the fifth on ways his homeland might safeguard its state by land and sea, and the sixth on

---

12 Cornaro, despite his denial, remained upset over this loss. See "Intro.," p. 41.

the way Venice can become stronger and more beautiful with increased revenue.[13]

He was a man loving and calm, nor did he ever quarrel with anyone, not lacking in generosity, which was the greatest and that he demonstrated in his youth; for when he was called upon to be generous he showed it. He had numerous friends because he loved everyone, and would help everyone as long as he could. And to remain helpful even after his death, he pledged his body to be opened and make known how well a sober life had conserved him inside overall.[14] He wanted his body to be buried with the bones of several of his friends and he did not want a showy funeral.[15]

---

13 Of the six works, three are known: *Aquae* (1560/64), *Architettura* (1547/54), and *La Vita Sobria* (1558). See "Intro.," p. 6–7, 8n12.

14 The study of anatomy was very important in Paduan teaching, "especially from 1537 when Andrea Vesalio was made the Chair of Anatomy and Surgery: his revolutionary *De humani corporis fabrica* appeared in 1543 and the second edition in 1555. Great anatomists to follow Vesalio were Realdo Colombo, author of *De re anatomica* (1559), Gabriele Falloppio, and Fabrizio Acquapendente, to whom the construction of the anatomical theatre at Palazzo del Bo is owed," *Scritti ...*, p. 134n12.

15 It is not known if this occurred. According to Milani, the location of his remains – as well as those of Angelo Beolco (Ruzzante) and Giovan Maria Falconetto, the two friends with whom he wished to be buried – is still unknown. See "Intro.," p. 69.

Selected Letters

LETTER FROM MESSER SPERON SPERONI[1] TO HIS MAGNIFICENCE ALVISE CORNER

[discourse against sobriety]

Your letter is one of approval of me because it is a sign that you remember me with love, and that you care about my life. And it is also one of enormous disapproval when, according to you, I am doing what is harmful and shameful to myself, for which you reprimand me. So then, in part I thank you, and in part I must justify myself, and if I cannot or do not wish to amend my ways, at least through words, it will thus not seem that my none sober life – in which many others, rather, nobles, keep me company – is lacking a defender in addition to be lacking in praise. But I would like to begin this defence against threats. Your Magnificence must have read of Asclepius,[2] son of Apollo, who was so excellent a physician that he not only healed the ill but could also resuscitate the dead, as he did with Hippolytus. Concerning this, Pluto and the Parcae protested to Jupiter, saying it was not licit even for the gods much less for the sons of gods to resuscitate the dead, and if he [Asclepius] were to continue with it, Pluto would lose his jurisdiction not only for himself but for all the gods, since mortals

---

1 Sperone Speroni degli Alvarotti (1500–1588), highly regarded by the best minds of his time for his erudition, was a "great philosopher," accomplished orator, author, scholar (*Delle lingue*), playwright, on friendly terms with princes and popes.

2 Asclepius, a healer, was the deified mortal son of Apollo. After his death, the Romans supposedly brought him back to life, during a plague outbreak, embodied as a serpent. He was later symbolized encircling a wooden staff, and was adopted by medical associations such as the World Health Organisation (WHO). Two serpents climbing a winged staff, on the other hand, is a caduceus – the magic wand of the Greek Hermes or Roman winged Mercury, messenger of the gods, creator of magical incantations – often (erroneously) used as a medical symbol. The caduceus represents hermeticism, alchemy, occult arts, and the like. See for example Edward Tripp, *Crowell's Handbook of Classical Mythology* (New York: Harper Collins Publishers, 1970), pp. 107 and 143.

would then become equal to them in their resurrection [immortal].
For this reason, Jupiter acted to punish Asclepius and struck him dead.
Therefore, Your Magnificence, beware of this end, that with your art
you do not favour men against Pluto and the Parcae, as had Asclepius;
and though you may believe you will die by resolution, you may instead
be struck down by lightning. Nor does it serve to say – I teach how to
live, not how to resuscitate – since the difference is in the words not in
the effect. Rather, I would say to resuscitate is worse than what Asclepius
did, who resuscitated only one life, and you resuscitate all of a sober
life, with which all men would resuscitate themselves. Thus, you should
know that when Jupiter, Neptune, and Pluto divided up the world, to
Jupiter befell heaven and as a result human life, and thus our soul,
comes from Heaven; and to Neptune befell the sea, and to Pluto, Hell.
Over these divisions, Neptune and Pluto protested: Neptune protested
because no one navigated the seas, and so he was the god of fishes and
nothing else; Pluto protested because at that time people lived to nine
hundred, a thousand years, and so there was much solitude in Hell.
Jupiter was content if men were to become crazed and began to die,
though not on earth but in the sea, and this was to Neptune's satisfaction. [Jupiter] also wanted our lives shortened, but not being able to do
so with a sober life, he decided to strike down – not Asclepius, though
in the name of Asclepius – the sober life, and so made it extinct. Hell
then immediately became more populated than earth and soon the
dead were more numerous than the living. Therefore, your Magnificence, if you were to resuscitate the sober life, the troubles of the world
that once were the despair of the world would return and again reduce
it to that chaos, from which may the Lord God keep us all safe. And I
remember having read that men, I refer to the sages,[3] complained to
Jupiter about this harm done to the human race for having shortened
life in this way by killing off sobriety; and that they at least, if not the
common people, wished to return to living those many hundreds of
years that were lived at the time of Methuselah. But Jupiter told them
that a sentence once made could not be changed, nor, reasonably
speaking, should it be changed, and that he marvelled at these sages, by
profession men of reason, who, contrary to reason, were procuring to
live longer, and that in their desire of this, they were more sensual than
the common person, *and quite lacking in judgment. And he proved

---

3 A person of rare and profound wisdom, prudent and judicious.

this in saying that if they alone were to have a long life, and common
people a short one,*◊ it would then be worse for them, because the
worst thing is to live too long having to watch, by living too long, the
death of their dearest brothers, sons, and friends, who were not as
knowledgeable. It would thus be a form of cruelty, and a sign of little
love for those close to them and of their presumption against God, to
Whom they had hoped to liken themselves by living long and by learning a great deal; and that their knowing too much was in vain, because
to oversee a world full of ignorance it is enough to know a little, not
a lot, and a little can be learned in a short time. A sober life, Jupiter
continued, was destroying medicine; therefore, a sober life gives rise to
ignorance of the countless beautiful natural things that are the properties of herbs, roots, flowers, and waters, since the sober life was always
thinking about eating, which then detracted from the many other beautiful and virtuous thoughts and works. So that, if a sober life commands
one to eat just so much – no more and no less, and only those things
and at that time and no later or no taking longer – then one need
never fast, nor ever do anything that might interrupt this order: not
study, not walk, and not fight for your country. Because doing so would
interrupt the order of foods, and the quantity of them, and the time for
eating them; hence, whoever studies and sits, digests less than the one
who fights and walks. It destroys virtue and above all that of strength,
which *in infirmitate proficitur*,[4] and it does away with justice, which is to
give to each thing that which belongs to it. But the sober life thinks of
nothing but its eating and even wants to take from death that which
belongs to death, which is portrayed with a scythe that can slice but not
resolve. A fine thing it would be, at the time of advising and fighting for
his country, to see the wise man eat his meal, for which more abomina-
ble would be the eating of it than the weighing of it. Nor are those the
scales of sobriety but of justice. ♦**It will not be a Christian thing, since
good Christians will never think about eating, that is, not about the

---

◊ Text between asterisks (*) was inserted by Milani to indicate a passage found in the
copy of the letter among the Speroni manuscripts (Biblioteca Vescovile di Padova
(T.XI), but not found in the Codex Vienna copy). See *Scritti ...*, p. 207.

4 *Virtus in infirmitate proficitur*, in II Corinthians 12:9, "my strength is made perfect in
weakness," *NKJV*.

♦ [Two passages inserted by Milani, shown here between double asterisks (**), were
found in the copy of the letter among the Speroni MSS (Biblioteca Vescovile di Padova (T.XI) but not in the Codex Vienna copy. See *Scritti ...*, p. 207.]

timing nor the quantity or quality of their food; but wherever they eat, they will eat what is placed before them, never bringing anything with them either to eat or drink.** And this sober person will always want his flask with him, not differing in this from the Germans, except that the German will have more.[5] **The good Christian will differentiate his time and this sober one his food; but now let us leave the Christian, who is still to become [sober] but is not yet, and let us speak logically.** The sober one has emotions that are in vain since he does not satisfy them; it would be better to satisfy the senses than to satisfy life, because the senses are nevertheless noble, being only in animals and in men, while life is also found in plants. The sober one will thus be more tree than man, but worse than a tree, because a tree always feeds itself, the sober one instead does not. It is quite true that just as a tree does not complain, so too the sober person will not complain, but down here never complaining is deficiency or stupidity, just as in Heaven where the contrary [to complain] is not good sense.

So it is that one should never eat unless it is to live. Is everything then to this end? Is friendship as well? And riches? And power? And science? Health, according to good philosophers, is a great good but not the ultimate [good],[6] nor is pain the worst that one could have. Worse yet would be to ignore his duty to friends, to posterity, and to country, all of which of necessity is ignored, if to live long in good health is our end purpose. But what can I say about health? The sober life cannot be called healthy, because health is an accident that together with its contrary, infirmity, mutually drive out one another from their subject. Therefore, if in a sober life there can be no infirmity, [then] there can be no health, and I am speaking of that true health, according to which we operate as wise men. And if we eat just enough to live on and no

---

5 Speroni may be referring to the *landsknechts* (lansquenets), mercenary soldiers, originally formed by Maximilian I of Austria in 1493 (and instituted elsewhere in Europe between the 15th and 17th centuries). Though fashioned after the Swiss mercenaries, they were a separate force, which was named not for their lances but for the German words meaning "land (country)" + "servant" (*knecht*), as they first served in the lowlands of the Holy Roman Eastern Empire. They fought battles at Ravenna and Pavia and were infamous for their violent acts during the 1527 Sack of Rome.

6 A possible reference to *summum bonum*, Latin for the highest or ultimate or supreme Good. A classical notion regarding that which "human beings, it is supposed, pursue by their very nature." (*Cambridge Dictionary of Philosophy*, 2001, *s.v.*). Most typically a philosophical notion of monists, believing in a single good: for example, the "Idea" (Plato), or eudemonism (Aristotle), or oneness with God (Aquinas).

more, then we will not walk, we will not jump, and we will never fight; nor could we ever do so, because we would not have the strength while eating only enough to live on. This will be a great defect in man, since boys eat not only to live but to grow, and men not only to live but to procreate, and so, being old men, we should eat, if not to grow and procreate, at least to operate as humans in other ways.

To be sure, I believe many of these things to be true, and I am certain that just as a crippled hand is not a hand because it cannot operate otherwise, so too the sober life is not life but half-death, because it does not operate as much as or in the way a man should operate. And I believe that to die from resolution, which your Magnificence glorifies, is for a man the worst manner of death possible, because it is to die from starvation; a death that Homer – speaking through the friends of Ulysses – infinitely despises, and he elects to drown them rather than have them starve to death. Nor does Dante blame the Pisans for any other reason than for making Count Ugolino die from starvation, even if he was a traitor to his country.[7] Moreover, to die from resolution is troublesome not just for the one who dies in this way, but also for the one who sees him die in this way. In regard to which, we can, for example, discuss the death and extinction of a candle out of resolution, which is troubling to everyone; because first it burns and then it does not and then hisses and seems to cry out, at which point, unable to tolerate this, gentlemen have it taken away rather than allowing it to finish, and they get another one. There would then be the danger that seeing a man die from starvation out of resolution – with a man being more valuable than a candle – it would greatly trouble the one to watch him die; thus the danger that he be buried before having ended or that

---

7 Dante Alighieri (1265–1321). "Ah, Pisa, you the scandal of the peoples / of that fair land where *si* [i.e., Italian] is heard, because / your neighbours are so slow to punish you, / may, then, Caprara and Gorgona move / and build a hedge across the Arno's mouth / so that it may drown every soul in you! / For if Count Ugolino was reputed / to have betrayed your fortresses, there was / no need to have his sons endure such torment," Dante, *The Divine Comedy of Dante Alighieri: Inferno*. Intro., notes and trans. Allen Mandelbaum (New York: Random House, Bantam Classic, 1982): *Inferno* XXXIII: vv. 79–87. In contrast to Speroni, Robert Hollander observes: "Dante's apostrophe of Pisa, 'new Thebes,' blames the city, not for killing Ugolino, which it had reason to do (if not perhaps a correct one), but for killing the children. All of Dante's sympathy is lodged with the children, none with Ugolino," *Dante: The Inferno*, Intro. and notes Robert Hollander, trans. Robert Hollander and Jean Hollander (New York: Doubleday, 2000), p. 571, note on vv. 79–90.

he be strangled out of compassion. And here, to confirm what I have said, I call upon Caesar, who chose to die an unthinkable death, which is not that of resolution, something foreseen and irremediable, because there is no remedy for resolution as there is for pain or fever. Thus, it is better to choose, it being unavoidable, to die like a man and not like a candle, so that the sober life, which leads us to such a death, is to be avoided like the plague, or better still, like hectic fever, or consumption, or dropsy. Even though your Magnificence remains happy and sings and laughs more than other none sober persons, I do recall, however, seeing you very much bent over, the result of your bones over drying, which are lacking in the humour and strength to remain upright; and this is due to the sobriety that dries up their radical moisture, since it does not have to dry up the unnatural [presence] of food. In short, he who is sober about food, since it is not for food alone we live, must be sober in many other things, and in all of things be sober, that is, measured. And if we weigh the wine and bread, and count the hours, we should also weigh thoughts, writings, readings, and those things that impede our digestion, and count the meals and words that help digestion, and not sleep if not for a certain number of hours a day, and a certain number at night. All things that, as a rule of life, would become tedious to hermits and be odious to everyone, and whosoever were to practise it would be ostracizing himself on earth and in Heaven, for no one would want him in their life. Too much of a rare thing and too unusual, too affected and too vile is this sobriety, and too beyond reason; the world itself does not want it for its system nor its governing. And still at times it rains more than it should, like in deluges, and at times it is too hot or too dry like in the days of Phaëton.[8] At times the seas and rivers flood the earth, at times water cannot be found, at times the air moves so little it is still, at times not only does the earth tremble

---

8 In Greek mythology, Helios (Sun god) indulged his newly acknowledged son, Phaëtōn, by allowing him to drive the Sun-Chariot (Fire). But being inept, Phaëtōn first sent the untrusting horses rising up to scorch the sky (producing the Milky Way), then plunged to earth, setting it ablaze. To save the world from total destruction, Zeus struck Phaëtōn with a thunderbolt; he fell into the Eridanus river and died. His sisters, the Heliades, stayed weeping on the banks of the river, where they turned into "poplars and their tears into amber." Cycnus, King of Liguria, was a musician and a relative, who, having failed to save him, "mourned among the poplars," and "was transformed, becoming a swan." Hence, swans about to die sing a sad song. See for example, E. Tripp, *Crowell's Handbook ...*, p. 470.

but it opens up and shifts from side to side. And this is not disorder
but the marvellous order of things mutable, which should not be immutable. The earth when corrupted is not resolved but turns into her
contrary, as do other elements. And do we, being composed of those
elements, wish to be resolved into them? Heaven still moves and its
motion is always new from day to day, and it never was nor ever will be
the same; the moon now waxes now wanes, now sooner and now later,
waxing and waning. As for us, do we always want to exist by one rule of
life and measure it and regulate it as the years pass? Years do not make
us live even though they measure our life, for the old can be robust
and the young be frail; nor is our life in the regulating and weighing of
food, but in the exercising of our body and our spirit [*animo*] that we
conserve ourselves, and [just as exercising virtue resolves the bad humour of vice,][9] so too exercising the body resolves the bad undigested
humours – and in this resolution one becomes stronger, not weaker –
so too each day the sober life makes one weaker but never stronger nor
more vigorous.

Your Magnificence will say that I do well to defend disorder, living
disordered [as I do], which my leg can attest. My response is that it is
enough for me to live more soberly than a man in Rome,[10] and without
need of a back brace for a man of my age, and may God grant that in
me the pain that should go to my head alone should all go to my legs.
But what would you say if I were grateful for this pain in my leg, which
spares me from having a thousand other ills? It is certain that this is
so, nor by this do I wish to justify myself by showing others a way to
spare me from doing things that, being very healthy, I could not on my
honour refuse. Nor can I, without prejudice to my honour and to my
life (should my doctors ask) change such an old habit of living, even if
changing it were for the better; and the proof of this is in the life led by
Pope Clement under advice of Corte, which caused him to die.[11] I am
almost sixty-two years of age, and your Magnificence began to regulate

---

9 Insertion between square brackets follows the findings by Maria Rosa Loi in *Speroni Lettere ...*, (1994), p. 132.

10 Speroni may be alluding to Bishop Cornelio Musso, dedicatee and devotee of the *Vita sobria*, with his close ties to Rome under Pope Pius IV (1499–1565). The same pope who was criticized for maintaining an ongoing culture of austerity.

11 Matteo Corte was the physician to Pope Clement VII (Giulio de' Medici), who himself may have "died of stomach cancer in 1534." See *Scritti ...*, p. 211.

his life at the age of forty. Habit is a great thing, and just as whoever was
to impose disorder on you now would kill you, so too whoever was to
impose order on me now would kill me. Nothing in the world is more
disordered than the motion of errant stars,[12] – hence they are said to
be errant, that is, wandering – which possess neither certain motion
nor certain stillness; *and perhaps errant means mistaken but in any
case their being errant conserves,*[13] and perhaps for this they make
the world beautiful. Writing after meals, your Magnificence should
remember, is healthy for you, or at least it does no harm to you, but for
me it would be harmful;[14] hence you do it and I do not. On this, which
is eminently clear, I will say nothing more and conclude that many philosophers and a great many saints died young, who, on the other hand,
did not have to live less than soberly, while many wicked and ignorant
carnal persons arrived at one hundred years, to where – so God
may grant me the happiness of my blood [family] and my friends –
I would not like to arrive dying the way they do. Therefore, I will not
kill myself nor will I do anything where nourishment would operate to
kill me, but I will live far removed from this desire and from this cure
[of a sober life]. If Count Zan Iacomo has died it very much grieves
me for he deserved to live; but perhaps he would have died in more
glory twenty years ago.[15] May God grant him paradise, and conserve
your Magnificence, and me, and those who love us, each in his order
or disorder of living, though I have more of your order in my disorder

---

12 The seven errant planets or wandering stars. For Aristotle, stars were of two kinds,
    fixed or errant. At the time, all planets (and stars) including the sun, were thought to
    revolve around the earth.

13 The passage between asterisks (*) – according to the findings by M.R. Loi in *Speroni
    Lettere ...*, (1994), p. 132 – should be included, but it is missing from Milani's citation
    of this letter in *Scritti ...*, Lettera XXIV pp. 205–12.

14 For example, (Fauno's) Ficino (*De le vite ...*, 16*r*) instructs: "Si dee fuggire, che per
    due o tre hore doppo mangiare, non ci poniamo su qualche difficile speculatione, o
    a molto intentamente leggere," [One must avoid, for two or three hours after eating,
    undertaking any challenging speculation, or reading very intently], *Scritti ...*, p. 112n7.
    "Thinking itself disturbs the digestive process, which is why studying after a meal is
    absolutely forbidden. ... Excessive study also exhausts the body, leaving no energy left
    for processing food," while "gluttony is obviously lethal to the intellect." On the role
    of emotions on one's well-being at the table, see K. Albala, *Eating Right ...*, pp. 138–43.

15 The Count of Monte l'Abate, Gian Giacomo Leonardi (1498–1562), was a military
    engineer and ambassador for Francesco Maria della Rovere, the Duke of Urbino and
    Sora.

than you have of mine in yours. *But it pleases me*◊ that you have no disorders to bother you, for I am a grateful slave to them. I will write about myself in some other way to your Magnificence, who, loving me as you always have, will be happy for my good and saddened for my ills, on which – be it one or the other – I will write, depending how my fortune goes. But I cannot have any illness that might disable me and make me despair, nor good that might render me insolent; neither the former nor the latter will keep me from your Magnificence, to whom I commend myself.

Rome, day 22 of February 1562.

◊ Different again from Milani, according to M.R. Loi's finding of Speroni, this phrase, "Ma mi piace …," – translated in English between asterisks (*) as "But it pleases me" – should be included. See M.R. Loi in *Speroni Lettere …*, 1994, p. 132.

Sperone Speroni: Letter in Favour of Sobriety[16]

To the Same [Cornaro] [no date]

Your Magnificent Lordship,

We learn that Stesicorus the ancient Sicilian poet, because he spoke ill
of Helen the daughter of Jupiter in several of his verses, went blind.
But later, repenting for having spoken ill of her and by writing to the
contrary, his eyesight was returned. Now if this is what happened to him
for speaking ill and then speaking well of a woman undeniably beautiful – but whose beauty caused the numerous deaths of Trojans and
Greeks, Scythians and Ethiopians, together with the ruin of so great a
kingdom – should I not believe that something similar will happen to
me? In one of my letters I spoke ill of sobriety, which is either a virtue –
and among the important ones, the first – or a light and pathway leading directly to virtue and to God Himself. Certainly it conserves man
for a long time in an honourable life, which reconciles the appetite
with reason and the intellect with the faculties; and it is no less good
than beautiful, no less happy than serious. I spoke ill of it, and though
I did not go blind like that other one, surely in speaking ill of it I was

---

16 In a letter dated 11 April 1562 to Cardinal Capo Di Vacca, Speroni writes: "Credo che si-
ate certo che la lettera da me scritta al magnifico Cornero è tutta burla; e questo è quanto piacere posso sentire e far sentire a' miei amici. Ma tosto gliene mandarò un'altra di
pentimento e con questa cancellarò il peccato della prima." [Knowing you are sure the
letter I wrote [against a sober life] to the Magnificent Cornero is all in jest gives me as
much pleasure as I can feel and have my friends feel. But soon I will send him another
one of repentance, and with this cancel the sin of the first] (S. Speroni, *Speroni lettere ...*,
v. 2, p. 135). For the above letter in praise of the sober life, see S. Speroni, ibid.,
pp. 254–6. This second letter in favour is not found in the Milani edition.

more blind than he, because I was blind in understanding, not knowing
how much I was sinning by writing such a wicked letter, and now, not
without the blessing of God, I believe I should retract it, and I believe –
unlike Stesicorus, after the fact – [it should be] before the moment has
passed and the good light of reason is taken away. Because not only do
I see my error, but I clearly see in this rare virtue all of its glories: and
if I am able to write about these as favourably as I see and discern them
in me, I hope to do no less glory for [sobriety] through my writing than
you do through your practise of it. Perhaps you will say I am like those
who praise acorns, since it is a food of the heroes, but do not enjoy
them; or that I am like those who are ill with gout and though com-
mitting every disorder think they will get better if they devote themselves to Saint Gotthard.[17] In reply I will tell you, in truth, my leg still
hurts me somewhat and I wish to heal it, but out of good conscience
I desire more to tell the truth and to praise the praiseworthy. And just
as you would like to have my illness to free yourself of it, being sure to
be freed of it through this blessed sobriety, so too I would be content
for the good of the world to die of this ill, if by my example the world
would then right its wrong. And what the world will not do for this
good – the good that comes from living a sober life – it may do for the
ill, which may come to me because of disorders. But come what may, I
will still do this and speak about this good, which I feel in my soul and
I am committed to speak about the sobriety of life.

Sobriety truly is either one and the same as temperance – one of the
virtues we should have – or it is the perfection of temperance and, just
like it, the magnificence of generosity and the magnanimity of fortitude. Temperance mixes wine with water, but sobriety, going further,
rather, ascending higher, drinks little of that mixture. Therefore, sobriety is a virtue more divine than human, being the perfection of human
[virtues] and not then of temperance, but of all the others.[18] And this

---

17 Saint Gotthard (960–1038) of Hildesheim was a Bavarian monk who became abbot
and later bishop. He was canonized in 1131. He worked to establish schools and
hospices for the sick and indigent; his name was invoked against all manner of ills including "hailstones, the pain of childbirth, and gout." Having also become the patron
saint of travellers, a chapel was dedicated to him along a pass in the Swiss Alps known
as St. Gotthard's Pass.

18 One of the four cardinal Virtues (along with Justice, Prudence, Fortitude), Temperance (Continence) is defined as self-restraint and moderation over the appetites;
self-control over excessive (superfluous) eating or drinking, or sex (even to the point
of abstinence), to temper the bodily humours and maintain their balance. See "Terminology": *Continence, Humours.*

– what we call *sobriety* – the ancients called *ne quid nimis* [no thing in excess], the sentence handed down to man from God as a great gift, if well executed, warning mortals of the need to live soberly in all their pronouncements.[19] And so it is – to leave aside what is already clear – that the one who knows too much scorns the world and by the world is loathed. The one too wealthy is envied, robbed, looted, and destroyed for his possessions; too much beauty is rarely demure, as in the example of the aforesaid Helen; the too powerful becomes arrogant and wages war on everyone; the too large is feeble of mind and the too small is ridiculed as a dwarf or pygmy. But let us end with this conclusion: that sobriety is the enhancement [*condimento*] of the virtues, of the sciences, and of every other good there is to be had down here and perhaps also up there on high. In truth, it is that the most beautiful angel in Paradise grew self-important because of his beauty, and on his own plotted to equal the Almighty; and if that harms our soul and the angels, which are pure spirit and immortal, how much will the absence of this holy sobriety harm our body and our mortal life? I said "will harm," I should say "harms," for not to live soberly still harms the one who lives that [other] way and is the cause of infirmity and death, as we see every day. I can say that the death of just one person very often gives rise to the ruin of a province: whereby the one who is not sober harms himself and the ones dearest to him and the people and the kingdoms. But let us now speak of infirmity.

I recall having read in St Basil that not fasting in accordance to the sober way[20] – that is, without limits and without discretion, hence,

---

19 The ancient site (c.1400s BCE) of the Oracle of Delphi was viewed as the exact centre or navel (omphalos) of the earth. A temple to Apollo (sixth century BCE) was later built, wherein the popular expressions: *mēden agan* (nothing too much), *gnōthi seauton* (know thyself), and *eggua para d'atē* (promise is allied to mischief), were alleged to be inscribed, though scholars today remain doubtful. Also see sophrosyne. Cf., Publius Terentius Afer (195/185–159 BCE), or Terence, a (Libyan?) playwright of the Roman Republic, "*Adprime in vita esse utile, ut ne quid nimis,*" (Excess in nothing, this I regard as a principle of the highest value in life), (*Andria* I, 1, 33) in W.G. Benham, *A Book of Quotations, Proverbs and Household Words* (London: Cassell, 1907), p. 556.

20 St. Basil the Great of Caesarea (330?–379), Cappadocian monk, Archbishop of Caesarea, came from a family with saints and martyrs. For Roman Catholics, his *On the Holy Spirit*, is the "definitive defense" of the divinity and consubstantiation of the Holy Spirit. The description of the monk's austere life: "His drink was water, his food bread and salt, his occupation labour and study" comes from F.W. Farrar's, *Lives of the Fathers: Sketches of Church History in Biography* (New York: Macmillan, 1889), p. 10. Deemed the original "Santa Claus" (of the Eastern Church), his feast day is the second of January.

without judgment – is a bad thing, because in so doing man kills
himself, as if he were to poison himself or to cut open his veins. And if
he does not kill himself, he becomes infirm, and from his infirmity is
born a contrary effect, contrary to what fasting intends to do; because
fasting is done with the clear intent of serving God, something that the
infirm cannot do. As someone infirm cannot go around here and there
exercising the office of charity toward his neighbour, he cannot go to
church and pray as he once did, nor take care of his family. Therefore,
if fasting – in itself a good thing – becomes evil when it is the cause
of many ills, what must be said of crapula, in itself bad, which is the
cause of all the above ills and countless others? Or, if contraries are
in themselves a science, and crapula, as we see, is the cause of our ills,
then sobriety – its contrary – is the cause of their contraries, that is, of
the good that are contrary to those bad. It will make us healthy, dutiful,
and useful to those at home and to all neighbours of our city, and dili-
gent in our duties; it will make the senses healthy in our body and calm
our thoughts. To this holy sobriety, Christ invited us, and he praised it
and implemented it while fasting in the desert, telling those who were
possessed to make themselves well through it and through prayer. The
Church also invites us to do this during Lent, the Fridays and Saturdays,
the four [seasons of] Ember Days[21] and the [three] days of abstinence,
whose solemnity often commands temperance from us, when it wishes
us to abstain from meat; at other times, temperance commands its
perfection – that is, holy sobriety – wanting as well that fish be eaten
less. And here I am reminded that I should speak to those who never
fast as commanded and that I offer myself [as an example] so as to give
them licence never to fast, but not so they stay as crapulent as before,
but so as to live soberly. By which I mean that if the world were to live
soberly, fasting would be superfluous, in the way certain philosophers
once said: that if there were friendship in the world, there would be no
need for justice. Saint John the Baptist lived on apples and locusts, and

---

21 An ancient heathen rite adopted by the papacy to attract converts (fifth century?) in
Rome. The Western Christian order of days, as later established by Pope (St.) Gregory
VII (1073–1085), consists of three prescribed days for fasting and prayer – during
each of the four seasons (*jejunia quatuor tempora*) – known as the Ember Days. They
consist of the Wednesday, Friday, and Saturday, immediately *after* the first day of
Lent, Pentecost (Whitsunday), the 14th of September (Holy Cross) and the 13th of
December (Santa Lucia). In 1966, Pope Paul VI excluded them as sanctioned days for
fasting.

it was he who heralded and led the way for Christ. '*Sobri estote*,' said the apostle,[22] and this word [sober] alone seems to promise every good. We men, not quite beasts, complain that life is short, not only in its too few years but in the little time of those few years, since at least one third of them is spent in sleeping – and I speak of a natural sleep. But I would add that crapula prevents us from living in two ways: the one is that we die sooner and the other is that, of the time we have to live, at least one half of it we sleep through. Sobriety, to the contrary, allows us to live more years and the major part of those years, that is, because of it, we sleep less. Thus, it frees us of sleep, which is half-death, thus, there is no difference between living happy or unhappy, and thus, it is the reason for our great happiness. If, when assailed from within and from without, one lives a sober life, people will better defend themselves and be better able in their offence. Man, therefore, being always assailed by infirmity and death, will better defend himself when sober than when full of food; and of that fullness, the poet says: '*Somno vinoque sepulti*,'[23] which is more than dead. He who eats little is closer to the angels who eat nothing, not to the devil who devours the sinner, '*Et semper quaerit quem devoret*.'[24] He sinned … .

----

22 Said by Peter: "sobrii estote vigilate quia adversarius vester diabolus tamquam leo rugiens circuit quaerens quem devoret" [be sober, be vigilant; because your adversary the devil, as a roaring lion, walketh about, seeking whom he may devour], I Peter 5: 8, *NKJV*.

23 The full phrase in Latin is "vino domiti somnoque sepulti" [o'ercome with wine and buried in slumber], Virgil, *The Aeneid of Virgil.* Ed. with intro. T. E. Page (London; Toronto: St. Martin's Press and MacMillan & Co. Ltd., first edition 1894, 1962), II, p. 265 and p. 228.

24 I Peter 5: 8, [And always searches for someone he may devour]. See above, note 22.

II

To Messer Luigi Cornelio in Padua

It pleases me, my dear Messer Luigi, that you would think of undertaking to help me. For in truth, your wanting to give me a good administrator means to help me a great deal, since I have need of one, as you know. But these times, so full of mistrust because of the plague, make me think only of taking care of myself and of removing from around me any reason to work with others, except with my own. Therefore, you will have to content yourself to let pass that menacing cloud now over us,[25] and then most willingly I will think about what you have written to me. And if your Novellino is as you believe him to be,[26] I will gladly make you happy on that account. In the meantime, guard well against misfortune, and live happily together with your good and most kind Messer Agnolo;[27] I envy you both a great deal. Be in good health.

4 July 1528. *Di Villa* [at the villa].

Pietro Bembo[28]

---

25 Famine occurred in the Veneto in 1528, and in the summer there was a "petechial" typhus epidemic, which spread throughout Europe.

26 According to Milani, "Novellino," about whom nothing else is known, refers to an estate administrator proposed by Cornaro to Bembo (*Scritti ...,* p. 140n3).

27 Angelo Beolco or Ruzzante (or Ruzante), see p. 135n9.

28 Pietro Bembo (1470–1547) was a renowned Venetian poet, scholar, and cardinal. His thought and influence on literary (Tuscan) Italian is deemed critical to its development. He is also credited with the development of the 16th century madrigal in music. His father was the eminent Bernardo Bembo (1433–1519), an ambassador and statesman in Venice.

III

To the Most Excellent Messer Speron, son of the Speroni (*Mss. Speroni*)[29]

Most Excellent Messer Sperone, you who know many things and every day discover something and know the cause and reason for them, find for me what I look for and you will make me happy. I search for some way to have my friends believe that the bodily disorders that men have, cause these men to die young; I tell them this but they do not believe me. And even if not from disorders, they die and leave me in this misery where I find myself, and even more so after the death of our dearest Messer Ruzzante, which also would have killed me from extreme sorrow, if this could kill a man, and before my having reached the age of ninety. But it was not able, because order has made me immortal and has seen to it that at the age of fifty-eight I look to be about thirty-five years old;[30] and every day this order makes it possible for one who is ill to regain his health through simple order. I say and I predicate each of these things every day but I am not believed, and this alone saddens me, for I could be the happiest man in the world. And so that you may believe me and undertake to find this remedy, for which you will then be my only God, you will hear of nothing else I need to make me happy. To begin with, I was born infirm, that is, with a weak

---

29 It is the best known letter by Cornaro for having been the most published, after Gamba had chosen it (1816) from among the Speroni papers. According to Milani, the published letter had been reworked with respect to the original, and the only ones who would later restore Cornaro's autograph text were Emilio Menegazzo and Claudio Bellinati, see *Scritti ...*, p. 141n1.

30 Cornaro is either fifty-eight or sixty in 1542. In his letter against a sober life (*Sober ...*, pp. 140–48, Speroni, assuming he knew Cornaro's true age, could have revealed it. Instead, as suggested by Milani, it was possible that he chose to go along with Cornaro's strategy. See *Scritti ...*, p. 98n21.

complexion and disordered; and having understood my condition, I
resolutely began to escape my disorders and so gained the great health
that is mine. For my family in my native land, I later acquired the use
of [our] nobility, which had been lost to me owing to [the oversight of]
my relatives; and it did not help that they had been great senators or
princes, for I regained the thing I was born without, even though my
relatives were very wealthy. And I regained it in the best way, a way more
worthy than any other, that is, by the means of blessed agriculture, and
not by armed means or by force and injury to others, nor by means of
crossing the seas with its infinite perils to life, or by other means full
of adversity. So it was that by one simple exemplary way I reclaimed
it – always combined with heavy expenses – and not by reducing costs
or the pleasures proper to a gentleman: things that elude someone
without wealth but who wishes to have them.[31] Yet, with that extensive
spending I have achieved it with a building of my own to God, a temple
built at my expense, giving to this God a following. I accomplished this
by having the foul air removed from inside that villa, where children
could not be raised; and in freeing it of those waters I brought countless people into the world. In gaining wealth, I have made many of my
administrators rich and many of my servants, and with my [wealth] I
have always helped writers, musicians, architects, painters, sculptors,
and others similar. In doing so, I have spent many piles and piles of
scudi[32] on a number of worthy constructions and on some of the most
beautiful gardens. And if I may, I can rightly call myself happy – this
you can believe – and I can say it is all for the three acquisitions already
mentioned, that is, with that of my health, that of nobility, and with
that of wealth – only by commendable means and justifiable expenses.
But there are still other reasons and motives as to why I am my happiest, which is that I have found and have a son-in-law – made especially
by Nature for myself and for my daughter – who is from the court, and
[together they have] three little children that are the epitome of three
little angels.

---

31 His daughter Chiara's marriage to Giovanni Cornaro Piscopia, who was a Cornaro
    noble, brought to her the long sought distinction of a noble surname ("Intro.," pp.
    55–6). Cornaro himself had been denied any claim to nobility by Venetian authorities.
32 *Scudo* was a large coin made of either silver or gold, so named for the shield (*scudo*) of
    the pontiff or noble issuing it; a pontifical *scudo* was first circulated in the late 1500s.
    A form of the *scudo* in Italy is said to have remained in circulation up until World
    War I.

And I enjoy these things in the best of health, in those comfortable
dwellings and those beautiful gardens, which are things I have accomplished. And the one who accomplishes these things can only enjoy
them, which I do enjoy and will enjoy for many more years. This being
so, as in effect it is, how is it I am not happy? I will be happy if you find
a way to dispose of that one opposition. And so that you do not think
there may be other obstacles to my happiness and that, without them
having been disposed, there could therefore be other ones (given that
every little conflict brings unhappiness), and since you know that piles
of money were taken from me in the matter of the Cardinal[33] – true,
against all reason much was taken from me – this, however, is not the
reason I am sad. Rather, it made me happy, because if this injustice
had not ensued, no one would have believed that, since I was good at
making estate administrators and servants rich, I could have made a
cardinal equally wealthy. Moreover, as you know, the officials overseeing
the waters caused me further notable damage, for which I assure you
I am similarly happy; because I would not otherwise have become the
liberator of our homeland, as I have become – because this injustice
was the reason I found a way for conserving the lagoon, and hence,
my homeland. Therefore, neither one nor the other of the above
can disturb my happiness, rather, they have allowed everyone to see
how strong and steadfast I am in the face of adversity, how astute and
helpful and happy I am in good times. It is something I was judged to
be the opposite, [something] considered almost impossible, since [to
others] I was always nothing if not most fortunate;[34] and yet despite
this, I made it known that I could turn wretched fortune into good.

---

33 Francesco di Alvise Pisani (1494–1570), was Cardinal and Bishop of Padua, and the
   Archbishop of Nardona. Supportive of Pope Clement VII, Pisani was held hostage
   for eighteen months by Charles V in Naples (1527 Sack of Rome). For many years,
   Cornaro had been an administrator for him in Padua, but after a dispute over
   Cornaro's management of the diocese revenue, they became embroiled in bitter and
   protracted litigation. In 1537 Cornaro entered further litigation over accusations that
   the embankments, which he and his partners had constructed, had contributed to the
   flooding of the lagoon. A formidable opponent to Cornaro was Cristoforo Sabbadino
   (1489–1543), who was made *proto* (Chief) engineer in 1542 for the Magistratura alle
   acque of Venice, and said to be a brilliant "hydraulic scientist." See for example, Manfredo Tafuri's *Venezia e il Rinascimento* (1985), trans., *Venice and the Renaissance* (1995).
34 A possible reference to Cornaro's inheritance from his father, and from his maternal
   uncle, Giacomo Alvise Angelieri.

And so to conclude, I have no other opposition to my happiness if not for the [premature] death of my friends, who die because they do not believe me and so keep me in continuing misery; thus, I pray that you act quickly for them.

And because I know how you have very much promised people that our Messer Agnolo [Ruzzante] will recite in your candid and admirable tragedy, and so that you do not think that you have also lost my favour, I am thus letting you know that I have no need of anything, and as I may come to Padua, which will be soon, I will see you, and I commend myself to you. Codevico, 2 April 1542.

Your Alvise Cornaro

X

Your Most Illustrious and Most Reverend Lordship[35]

Do not think sad thoughts of me, to where I know your kindness and charity lead you by thinking that I have reached the advanced age of seventy-six years, and now that the season is winter – so very adverse to the old – and since the past two winters I have been ill that I would therefore be so once again. Do away with that thought, Most Reverend Lordship, and be happy that I am healthy, having found the remedy against a winter in which I would have fallen ill; a proper remedy, reasonable and natural, which will still be beneficial to you when you arrive at this beautiful age.

It must be understood, Most Reverend Lordship, that the more the years increase for an old man, the more his strength and his stomach heat decrease and the more it cools; however, it is by the heat of summer and the strength of the sun that the warmth of that stomach is sustained, so that he may digest his usual food. But because the cold of winter has a contrary effect and the stomach cannot digest that same quantity, and the undigested part is converted into bad humours, which keep that old man indisposed and in the end makes him ill, and I, already feeling thus indisposed for two years, so as not to become ill, wished to reduce the amount myself. Yet, compelled by my family and friends, I consulted with doctors, who then concluded that the amount of food I would reduce was the amount of prosperity and strength I would be reducing in my body. Because my being indisposed comes

---

35 Written to Sperone Speroni, who was some sixteen to eighteen years younger than Cornaro.

from the accumulation of my years and not from too much food, they instead determined that for my body to sustain its strength, I should increase the amount. And so as not to appear more of a physician than they, and to please my family and friends, I increased the amount, with the result that in a matter of days I fell ill; and with an illness as great as my disorder had been great, whereupon I was judged to be a dead man by my doctors. And yet, by medicating myself – according to my own natural method, not to theirs – I regained my health, and with summer returning I increased the food to my usual amount. For the following winter I wanted to reduce it again but was discouraged by them, whereupon I once again fell ill, though much less seriously, since the disorder of not reducing my food was less than that of increasing it. But, so as not to fall ill a third time, I reduced it, and I am healthy; although, for the reasons stated by the aforesaid persons, I should with my increasing old age fall ill again and most gravely. I resolved to reduce the amount without further consulting with them, having understood that they do not know what to advise for an ordered and sober life. And it is most reasonable that they do not know – because their science is entirely founded on the disordered and on crapula – since the ordered has no need of either doctors or medicine but only of natural orders.

Therefore, be of good cheer, Most Reverend Lordship, that suddenly I have become free of the dangerous advice of doctors and of the illness, and do not fear, as the doctors foretold, that my strength was reduced in having my food reduced; rather, it has become greater, because this little amount of food all converts into perfect substance, just as that greater [excess] amount of food converted into bad. And since coolness will fall and warmth will rise, I will go on increasing my food [gradually] until I reach my usual amount; this will be my order for the next few years, but later I will be obliged to reduce it, because of nature and my increasing years. And I know that I will no longer make that error [of increasing food] – since it was because of it that I became ill – but I will stay healthy because I am most certain that Nature is content with little [food] in a body that has passed middle-age, and even more so if the body is old. But this goes unrecognized by those who are gluttonous and lacking in restraint [*incontinenti*], and who say that by reducing my food I made this error and harmed my sense of taste because I deprived it of its natural enjoyment, hence I will never taste the part that was reduced. To them we respond, it is a loss of so little importance that it goes unnoticed by someone who is continent; this person knowing that as food is passed along that short section of the throat, the less his taste [palate] is able to taste it, and that the moment it arrives there it is gone. Furthermore, it can be said that whosoever would not want to lose, for this reason, his sense of taste, should eat that little amount in the same time it would take to eat a large amount. He would then have this advantage: that, since it took a large amount to satisfy his sense of taste, [now] his taste will be satisfied by a little and he will taste with more subtlety. Besides, the one that eats little is assured it cannot harm him, just as the one who eats a large amount can be most assured that it will harm him. But beyond all the advantages cited above, there is this one great one, which is to be greatly appreciated, for the one who eats little, tastes plain bread more subtly than will the one who eats a large amount of a well-seasoned prepared dish created by the hands of a perfect cook. O what a truly subtle dish it is, Most Reverend Lordship, that of plain bread, accompanied by the natural desire to eat that comes from great health! And it is a most reasonable thing that this is so, bread being the proper and truly natural food of man, eaten by him as was said with a natural appetite arising from his health. It is true, Most Reverend Lordship, I give you my word, and it is so pleasurable to the taste that if it were not a natural and proper food of man, this food would be the sin of gluttony; our sense of taste [palate], as was said, enjoys so very much its taste.

This sense of taste, so perfect in man, is the result of an ordered and sober life and is one of its miracles, which is denied or disbelieved by those already mentioned, who are gluttonous and lacking in restraint [*incontinenti*], and who would never abandon their many and different foods to eat plain bread. And being miserable, they are unaware that such diversity, for various reasons, leads them instead to infirmities and to aging and then to death. This is because they are already old at the age of forty years and before they can reach fifty, they die. They do not deny this, rather, they admit they often become ill and at fifty years they die, but they say that this becoming ill and this dying does not come from eating different foods or from eating and drinking well, but by the powers of the Heavens and by chance and by destiny. And I who know from lengthy experience that they are greatly mistaken would like to let them know so they might live healthy and for a long time; and because I have pity for them, I say to them that a sober life is that very medicine so greatly praised – since it lets men live healthy and for a long time – which is called potable gold. [But the gold] is distilled to become a beverage, a medicine outside of Nature, therefore it cannot have a natural effect, as does sobriety, which is natural and is not alchemy.[36] In addition to convincing them through reason, which they cannot contradict, I tell them it cannot be denied that a disordered life is entirely contrary to that of an ordered one; thus, the one is the opposite and reverse of the other. Nor can it be denied that if the one has strength and power, then the other would have as much strength and power as its contrary; and that it cannot be said that a disordered [life] would not have great force, because it is a certain and commonly held thing. And whoever is of an age can attest the fact that after this disordered life and crapula were brought into our Italy by the French and was accepted by us, it operated by its own force; so that a man once old only at the age of eighty years – and who did not die until ninety or one hundred years – has now, as we see, become old at forty and may not live beyond fifty.

Similarly, the Germans die young, and yet they are born in a land with ideal air and well positioned by the Heavens, for which they are born with such good complexions – not only strong but robust and fierce – that they should live to and beyond the age of one hundred years and yet they die by the age of fifty. The only reason for this is crapula, which they have introduced by the force of a habit that has so much power it makes things that are against nature seem natural. And they do not realize, poor wretches, that it is not a virtue but a vice seeing themselves every day not in their right minds and not acting like humans but like animals. To be sure, Most Reverend Lordship, I am amazed at how they can be so strong and so fierce as to reach the age of twenty-five years while taking poison every day, which they take by overeating and drinking, whereby drinking more than necessary is only poison. And we recognize this only too well, as said, in their strange and foolhardy acts and the effects that it [crapula] has on them. Those same persons, gluttonous and lacking in restraint, cannot deny this much less what I am about to say – something they know to be true and certain – that at a tender age I was infirm owing to that disordered life, and with an ordered life I then regained my health and have remained healthy these thirty-two years. Since that time, I have fallen ill [in each of]

---

36 Cornaro was adamantly opposed to alchemy, evident in these writings, even though his own grandson Giacamo Alvise was an alchemist. Indeed, he omits any of his grandfather's comments against alchemy in the first collected edition he produced of the *Vita sobria* in 1591, see "Intro.,"pp. 32–4.

the past two years – for keeping a disordered life, on the advice of
doctors – because to increase my food was the greatest disorder for
someone so old, since I should have reduced it. And that it was a
disorder is seen this year, because I reduced [my food] and have not
been ill, though I should have been even more ill. Not able to refute
so many reasons and what can be seen as fact, they remain convinced,
but because they still do not wish to concede, they say that such a life
cannot be kept by a middle-aged man but only by an old man. The
disorders that disorder life are too many and too varied, and at least
one among these has the power to cause other disorders. And that one
[disorder] caused disorders in everything, since it is not possible that
man not suffer the heat, cold, fatigue, sun, wind or lack of his usual
amount of sleep. But even if he were to guard himself well against those
[disorders] and the many others, he cannot, however, guard against the
accidents of the soul, which are disorders; man cannot guard against
these and prevent them from causing joy or melancholy or anger within him. To them I respond that it is true they are all disorders, and fatal
ones, and that one disorder causes disorder in everything, but [only]
in a man so unregulated who does not maintain at least two orders in
his way of living. And it is not from the disorders noted above but the
ones I will name, which can be kept by each of us. One, is not to drink
wine nor eat food contrary to his stomach, and this can be done by
every middle-aged man; the other, is not to drink or eat except what his
stomach can digest with ease, and this again can be done by that same
man. By maintaining only these two orders – they alone having that
force and virtue – none of the many disorders above can make him ill,
because they do not have the force to generate bad humours in that
man's body as would the two [contrary] of the mouth above. With these
orders, a man may very well be left indisposed for one, two, or three
days, but they cannot make him ill with an alteration from fever, which
comes from the alteration of bad humours, which, as was said, cannot
exist in the body of one who leads a sober life.

And they – since they had finished with being gluttonous and lacking
in restraint [*incontinenti*] – having no response, say they are determined
to adopt that [sober] life; and to see that they will, I assure them it has
so much force and so much power in our bodies that if God had not
made our bodies mortal, sobriety would keep them alive to spite death.
And its force is known, because we see that it has the strength to liberate man from mortal infirmities, in the way it has liberated me. And if it
has such force to liberate him from those [infirmities] and from death,

producing his good health, so it should be believed – while he still maintains good health – that it would have as much force not having to fight infirmity and would thus keep him alive to spite death. But it cannot do this, because by the Will of God it is necessary that man die. But having to die, it is to his great advantage to die at the oldest age he can, in order to enjoy, in addition to the many other benefits, the beneficence of Nature. [Nature] produces a man so he may grow old and not die young, given that such a [disordered] man will enjoy neither mature age nor old age, which are the most important ages. The old man enjoys all ages; dying therefore is not troublesome to him as it is to the young. And he is beyond being troubled, because an old man, seeing himself at that advanced age – to where, out of a thousand born [only] one will not arrive – he calls himself content and satisfied with his long life. And he sees that death cannot trouble him, because once having reached a mature age he abandoned to that [youthful age] his sensuality, greed, and lack of restraint [*incontinenza*]; and in place of those vices he acquired sacred reason, useful continence, and exemplary prudence – the very virtues that for many years protected and safe-guarded him from his wrongdoings and sins. And though he may recognize himself as a sinner, he has made this vital acquisition: that he cannot fear the sorrows of that other life, having, as we said, abandoned wrongdoings; and having come to the most certain knowledge, after a long life, that Jesus Christ shed His precious blood for us, His Christians, and with that He liberated us from that sorrow. Moreover, he is liberated of the three human passions, which afflict a man so greatly, that is, from the ambition of honours, from avarice, and from lust, as well as from the two perturbations.[37] And he will have this advantage, that, since that body through sobriety is liberated of bad humours, his brain, therefore, being similarly purged through sobriety, is not harmed by any fumes from the stomach; and so purged he is liberated of wicked thoughts, and thinks only of otherworldly and lofty things, and so they are all lofty and spiritual. It should thus be concluded that the great grace and singular benefit is in the attainment of old age, but in good health.

We cannot reach this kind of old age if not by means of the ordered life discussed above. And it is quite true that some grow old not through those means but owing to their perfect complexion; yet,

---

37 The fear one develops of suffering in old age and the fear of impending death.

such persons are subject at every age to infirmities, and they are full of backaches and pains; because they did not know nor did they ever think about an ordered and sober life, but depended solely on their strong complexion. Therefore, when having passed a mature age, they did not abandon their sensuality and appetite, in this way taking away that place from reason and continence, without which man is unable to liberate himself of his infirmities and from thoughts of death and suffering, in addition to the three passions of man and from the two perturbations. Those who have reached that age are liberated of many of these contraries by following a straight path, as was demonstrated, and who, in living virtuously, always remain healthy and enjoy this beautiful world; which is truly beautiful for the one who knows the way to make it beautiful, as I know that you, Most Reverend Lordship, are capable of doing. And so it will not trouble you at this young age to think about old age, rather it brings happiness, your being most certain to enjoy, at that [old] age, the beauty of the world as I do. And because once arrived at that age you can take shelter from winter, I wished to do this for you and to show again my reverence by kissing your hand.

[Alvise Cornaro]

XIII

To the very Magnificent my Lord and Father his Lordship Luigi Cornaro
The Very Magnificent Lordship and Father.

What a sweet and dear letter this was from you! How well you have sweet-
ened this ill-fated but false news of my death! How very compassionately
you have interpreted it – that I might die by remaining in Bitonto! And in
the end, as you intimated in such a beautiful manner with your real and
true illness of actually having arrived at death's door, in no way therefore
should I regret this or be troubled over my being dead in name only! On
this your mortal infirmity – may the Lord bless – with the many wonderful clever remarks by which you describe it to me, and so by the love and
regard I have for you, not only does it not trouble me, but it truly does
amuse and delight me! But come now, you have always stood apart from
other men, as you are now and as you will be; nor after your death will
you ever die, but to spite death when you are dead you will live immor-
tally. And I will force myself to continue following in your footsteps, still
endeavouring, while Our Lord God grants me life, to live healthy, con-
soled by friends. On anything further, your Lordship will hear from our
Giuseppe, who I commend to you. Naples, 20 December 1556.

Giovanni Battista kisses your hands.[38]

May Your Lordship ensure that Giuseppe not leave, because I will soon
be arriving nearer to you, and each day you will know of everything.

Your son, Brother Cornelio,[39] *Bishop of Bitonto*

---

38 *Giuseppe ... Giuseppe*: Giuseppe Pavani was Chancellor to Musso; Giovanni Battista
   may have been a relative of Cornaro; perhaps G. Abriani, a "faithful servant" always
   remembered by him, see *Scritti ...*, p. 173n3.
39 Cornelio Musso. See *Sober ...*, p. 3n1.

Most Magnificent Lordship

I do not believe a more trustworthy testimony can be found, which cannot be contradicted – that sobriety is what makes a man happy in this life – than the testimony of Holy Scripture we can read in the first chapter of Daniel. Here, it prophetically recounts that having conquered Jerusalem, Nebuchadnezzar had a number of boys selected of noble, rather royal, blood, to be nurtured and educated as royalty, with the objective that they then be loyal to his person; and among these was Daniel, along with various others. It was thus on order of the king that these so chosen were to be nurtured only with royal foods, and liberally [generously] and royally educated, whereby after a period of three years they may be presented to the king in all their beauty and best refinement, being in effect – royal.

Daniel, feeling and knowing sobriety to be the only thing in this life that we must serve, as the fount of every virtue and perfection, pleaded with his governor not to feed him or his three companions – Hananiah, Mishael and Azariah[40] – any royal foods or delicacies,[41] but to nourish them right away with legumes and water; because their desire was living soberly for the health of their bodies and of their souls. Upon hearing

---

40 Daniel 3: 1–30. Shadrak, Mishak, Abednego (in Hebrew: Hananiah, Mishael, and Azariah) were from Israel, descended from nobles, who were brought to the courts of Nebuchadnezzar. In deference to the monotheism of their Jewish faith, they refused to bow down to the idol of the king, provoking his wrath. They were ordered to be thrown into the fire, from which they were confident they would be protected by God, and so emerged unscathed.

41 A delicacy was food that was "delightful" or delectable to the palate (taste), a term applied to refined, complexly flavoured, or unusual, foods.

this, his governor said: "God does not Wish me to disregard the royal mandate I have been given, and especially in this, so that by not feeding you [royal] delicacies, and after the mandated three years when you must be presented before the king, you could be, because of that sobriety, consumptive and less handsome, something that can bring injury and blame to me or even death."

Having heard why the governor would not ever [agree to] such a thing, under any circumstance, Daniel hastily stated that this could never happen, telling him: "I pray you, do this experiment for ten days and keep in mind that we will look better and have better colour than any of the others under your care who feed on delicacies."

So it was that the governor, convinced by this argument for experimentation, for ten days gave them the meals of the sober diet they had requested. When they appeared before him, he indeed found that Daniel and his companions were in far better form and well fed – through sobriety – and more attractive than those who had eaten sumptuously and royally in following the precept of the king. Hence, they continued for the next three years with that [sober] food.

And when all the boys who had been selected appeared before King Nebuchadnezzar, Daniel, together with his three said companions, were found to be the most beautiful of all the rest, with no comparison, and ten times superior to all the visionaries and learned men of Egypt; thus, this sobriety caused not only the body to be beautiful but also the soul and infinite knowledge. In Daniel, it also caused prophecy, because it was Daniel who not only interpreted the king's dream, but also revealed its secret – which had been forgotten [by the king] – about a statue, and thus saved the lives of all the learned men, who, by royal decree, were set to die for not knowing either how to reveal or how to interpret that dream or vision.

And it appears that Dante, at the end of canto 22, *Purgatory*, wished to celebrate it, praising and exalting this sobriety when he says:

... Et Daniello
dispregiò cibo, et acquistò sapere.

Later, the same Dante, at the beginning of canto 4, *Paradise* – speaking about the solution Daniel gave for the dream – said:

Fessì Beatrice qual fe Danïello
Nabuccodonosor, levando d'ira
che l'havea fatto ingiustamente fello.[42]

Now, these are the admirable results of the much praised sobriety, which
I observed not long ago, as its truest and wisest information and knowledge have helped me a great deal, and are helping; so that, in truth,
I can claim to be completely renewed in the health of my body, mind
[*mente*], and soul. Not particularly wanting at this time to explain the
benefit received – which, perhaps not ungratefully, will later be known
at a better time – all in thanks to this blessed sobriety; which, in the end,
like a most faithful companion, leads [health] not only to a spirit of
prophecy but also places it back in Heaven. This is similarly affirmed by
Philo Judaeus,[43] considered by all as the second Plato, and of course the
Magnificent Bartolomeo Zacco had also discovered such an authority in
Philo. And for this we should remain hopeful that [Zacco] may yet join
the school of sobriety, having been (as already known) as much opposed
to it; in so doing he will praise its wonderful brilliance and virtues to
Heaven, which, among the wise, is now celebrated throughout the world.

I will never cease from proclaiming the opinion of Epicurus[44] that it
has put an end to voluptuousness, so great is the fame of this sobriety
that being even more so is not possible. Here, in Latin, are his words as
we read from Diogenes Laërtius, the famous author:

> Itaque simplicibus, et no magnifice paratis cibis consuerscere et salubri-
> tatis efficiens est et hominem ad vitæ usus necessarios impigrum reddit.
> Magnificentioribus csi per intervalla sumantur, nos commodius aptat, atque
> adversus fortunam interritos facit.

> Cumque dicamus voluptatem finem esse unum summum bonum non
> luxuriosorum voluptates easque quæ in gustu sunt positæ, ut quidam

---

42   [And Daniel, spurned food and acquired knowledge] Dante, *La divina commedia*,
     trans. A. Mandelbaum, *Purgatorio* 22:145–6; [Then Beatrice did just as Daniel did, /
     when he appeased Nebuchadnezzar's anger, / the rage that made the king unjustly
     fierce], ibid., *Paradiso* 4:13–15.
43   Philo Judaeus of Alexandria (20 BCE–50 CE) is thought to have integrated Greek
     philosophy and Judaism.
44   Epicurus (341–270? BCE) was a Greek philosopher, born in Samos. A prolific author,
     his thought is now only known through surviving Herculaneum papyri (on nature),
     the epitomes (on physics, ethics, and astronomy), or through later followers – for
     example, as cited here, Diogenes Laërtius (third century CE), or in the first century

ignorantes aut a nostra sententia dissentientes aut male accipientes arbitrantur. Sed non dolere corpore animumque tranquillum esse, et perturbatione vacare dicimus. Non enim convivia et comessationes, non puerorum mulierumque congressus, non piscium usus et cæterorum, quæ affert preciosior mensa suavem gignit vitam, verum Ratio Sobria, causasque perscrutas, cur quæque vel eligenda vel fugienda sunt opinionesque expellens per quas animos ut plurimum occupat tumultus.[45]

Your Servant, P. P.[46] *(1558/9?)*

BCE with Philodemus, and Lucretius, though Cicero was critical of it. Very simply, the Hellenistic "Garden," Epicureanism, involves an earthly life of "pleasure," serenity, good friendship, and contemplation – free from political or religious constraints. This promotes *ataraxia* (a mind unperturbed and not fearful), and in the absence of bodily pain (aponia), it will maximize "pleasure" – an ideal of serenity of mind and higher thought over sensuality. As a modified (chance, or swerve) atomist, and believer in knowledge perceived through the senses, Epicurus did not hold to the immortality of the soul, and if sensation ceases when we die, then "Death is nothing to us"; therefore – as with the gods, who stay remote from man (remaining in their ideal "happiness") – death need not be feared. Epicurean thought – which "never entered the intellectual bloodstream of the ancient world" – was revived in the early modern era, reprising its rivalry with both Platonists and Stoics. Also see the "swerve" effect (clinamen in Lucretius) on free will and the study of physics.

45 Diogenis Laertii, *De vita et moribus philosophorum libri X,* (Lugduni: Eredi grifo, 1559), p. 461. [Again, we regard independence of outward things as a great good, not so as in all cases to use little, but so as to be contented with little if we have not much, being honestly persuaded that they have the sweetest enjoyment of luxury who stand least in need of it, and that whatever is natural is easily procured and only the vain and worthless hard to win. Plain fare gives as much pleasure as a costly diet, when once the pain of want has been removed, while bread and water confer the highest possible pleasure when they are brought to hungry lips. To habituate one's self, therefore, to simple and inexpensive diet supplies all that is needful for health, and enables a man to meet the necessary requirements of life without shrinking, and it places us in a better condition when we approach at intervals a costly fare and renders us fearless of fortune … When we say, then, that pleasure is the end and aim, we do not mean the pleasures of the prodigal or the pleasures of sensuality, as we are understood to do by some through ignorance, prejudice, or willful misrepresentation. By pleasure we mean the absence of pain in the body and of trouble in the soul. It is not an unbroken succession of drinking-bouts and of revelry, not sexual love, not the enjoyment of the fish and other delicacies of a luxurious table, which produce a pleasant life; it is sober reasoning, searching out the grounds of every choice and avoidance, and banishing those beliefs through which the greatest tumults take possession of the soul (Diogenes Laërtius on Epicurus in *Diogenes Laërtius: Lives of Eminent Philosophers,* trans. Robert D. Hicks (Cambridge, MA: Harvard University Press, 1925, rpt. 1995), vol. II: X, p. 655 and p. 657)].

46 P. P. is attributed to Paolo Pino, a Venetian painter, poet, and playwright, author of *Dialogo della pittura* (Venice, 1548), about whom "little else is known."

XVII

Draft of the letter written to Messer Zan Paulo da Ponte[47]

Day 1 of December 1559

Neither the death of my son-in-law, which leaves me with the great responsibility of being a father in his place to his eleven children, could diminish part of my generosity or a single particle of reason that is in me, nor the loss of an acquisition that I could have made of 150 thousand ducats[48] – lost to me because my women had little understanding of it – or for having lost the lawsuit selected to be overseen by them, contrary to my way of thinking.[49] So it is that all three of these

---

47 Zan (Giovanni) Paolo da Ponte, member of the wealthy da Ponte family, originally from 15th century Ferrara, lived in Venice. His granddaughter was Irene di Spilimbergo (1538–1599), a noted intellectual and artist. (The family name of Cornaro's wife was da Spilimbergo). A curious connection: the same Lorenzo Da Ponte (1749–1838), of this eponymous translation series, was born Emanuele Conegliano. He was about 14 years old when his widowed father, wishing to marry a Catholic, had the family convert from Judaism to Catholicism. Emanuele then took the name of the one who had baptized him – (Bishop) Lorenzo Da Ponte. This second Lorenzo Da Ponte (Emanuele) became a priest, opera librettist (for Mozart), and adventurer. He eventually absconded to the United States, where he later garnered fame as the first professor of Italian studies at Columbia (King's) College (now Columbia University). His good friend Piero Maroncelli (1795–1846), a writer and poet, wrote a not altogether accurate "Sketch of the Life of Cornaro," which was included in the 1842 (John Burdell) English edition of the *Vita sobria*. Da Ponte's second son, Lorenzo L. (1803–1840), was a professor (New York University) and collaborated on the work *Roman Antiquities: or an account of the manners and customs of the Romans* (1837); see "Bibliography": "Adam."

48 *ducat*: coin made of silver or gold. Existing elsewhere in Italy, the Venetian silver *ducato* was issued in 1202, the gold in 1284. The ducat standard was later adopted within Europe, remaining in circulation until the beginning of the twentieth century.

49 Cornaro corrected himself, replacing "happiness and contentment" with the more reliable "reason," (*Scritti ...*, p. 181n3). His wife and daughter had their own ideas

extraordinary and very damaging incidents had no power to diminish my spirit or my happiness or my contentment. For this blessing and miracle there must necessarily be a reason.

And here Lordship is the reason: that my having arrived at such an advanced age of eighty-five is thanks to my blessed Lady Continence and a prudent Ordered Life, from which was born my beautiful and agreeable health. Because these have completely removed the vice of the senses from everything and in its place put blessed reason. And with the senses no longer having force over me, but only reason, I am liberated from all accidents of the soul, and from passions and perturbations; thus, these three injuries could not sadden me. What is more, liberated of the unnatural death that results from infirmities and by living that [sober] life I have removed all causes of infirmity, and once removed, I removed that death. And I am confident and certain I can no longer die if not for a natural death, which is from resolution, once having passed the age of the one hundred years conceded and terminated by God, and by our own Mother Nature, to man, who does not overlook conserving his life as I have done. Therefore, my having many more years to live beyond the many I have lived, reason liberates me from that thought of death, as this no longer has a contrary sense; thus I live happily.

And to my happiness can be added these other causes. The first is that my grandchildren – in addition to their good health and their bodies not wanting for anything, being well formed and having good minds and kind natures, and being friends of virtue and enemies of vice – since they are rather well suited to letters, have gained a decent knowledge of them for their age. They are thus the sort, being young, to accomplish the things they set out to do, which is one of the many blessings available to these grandchildren of mine. This is the first cause, which adds happiness to my happiness.

The second cause is in seeing how well my practical advice – on the number of many undeveloped lands that may be cultivated, a most fine and important undertaking for the country – is about to succeed, because I had specified and advised on it so well. This has resulted in three great and practical benefits that account for my utmost

---

regarding his properties and legal problems, which may have contributed to his losing a lawsuit. According to Milani, Cornaro never really forgave them for making him forgo the "acquisition" (*Scritti* ..., p. 181n4 and p. 133n9).

happiness: the first is that the same undertaking gave life to more than twenty-five thousand souls, those among the unfortunate to be farm labourers, because – having already had three consecutive years of the Great Famine – if they had not had the work for earning a high wage, their children would have died, since they could not have made a living on their usual low wage. The second benefit is that the proprietors of those towns – the ones not utilizing those lands – who began cultivating, will have made a profit of 400,000 ducats on their income. The third benefit is that my homeland will make a profit from the ordinary taxation made on utilized lands and on yields from the crops growing there and other places; and this city, which had nothing to live on for ten months of the year, will have enough for fifteen. And these Euganean Hills instead – which were completely surrounded by swamps producing the foul air that has now been made good, and the mosquitoes that made the lands uninhabitable [now] no longer feed there – will have men of reason born there, and domesticated animals [raised].

These three benefits, for which I was the cause, I enjoy in my happiness, as I have said, and these are in addition to the benefit that I will achieve for my dear Homeland; which, to her great disadvantage has lost use of her port and a large part of her very important lagoon. But I have a way to restore the port and to be of much benefit in that.

Moreover, day by day there are new joys for me, since my treatise on the sober life, known throughout different places, has operated for the reasons now discussed, in as much as Germany has begun to ban excessive drinking. It is what men were doing by inviting each other [to drink] and viewing it as a virtuous [manly] act, when it is a dissolute and fatal one. Many of my friends and acquaintances from these neighbouring areas thank me, some by letter and some in person, for the useful guidance given them in that treatise. But persons who are often with me marvel at how, despite the passing of the years, my prosperity does not diminish nor does my happiness or my contentment. And they see that all my sensory capacities are ideal and that my brain is more of a brain than ever and my memory perfect, as are my teeth, but above all that my voice is more sound than ever and that my body is always free of pain or injury. Thus they conclude that these many and numerous benefits and blessings could not have come about if not for the sober life; as in fact is true. They therefore struggle to escape their senses and the vice of gluttony and to use far greater reason, which are things they are able to do, seeing that I myself have done them. And this adds to my happiness.

XXI

LETTER WRITTEN TO VARIOUS DUKES TO BE SENT WITH THE TREATISE OF THE SOBER LIFE[50]

Most Illustrious Duke

Being common opinion and truly reasonable that for kings, dukes, and others, who govern states – when good and courageous and when they beautify the world – and their subjects, and others, would therefore wish to live longer, and benefit and beautify the world longer. I myself have seen that there is a way to live for a long time always in good health up to the age of one hundred years: the term granted by God for the life of a man. And this is what God wishes for each of us to enjoy at each age, but above all at the oldest age, because it is the wisest, most honest, most liberated, and most religious of all other ages, the age that man enjoys infinitely. And as I said, having seen the way to attain that happiness and to demonstrate the way to do it, I have written this treatise that I am sending to your Lordship. It is not opposed by either doctors or philosophers but only by very sensual [persons], who do not however criticize it, and it is liked by those who read it. Nonetheless, they do make this objection: that it is not possible to do as much as it says because, as we know, it was not possible to institute the republic that Plato proposed in one of his treatises, which is beautiful to read but neither he nor others have ever been able to institute such a republic. And so it will be the same for my treatise, which wants a person throughout his life to maintain continence and a sober life, the enemies of the senses, of greed and gluttony; but these have such power over man that neither continence nor a sober life can be maintained.

---

50 Cornaro had written this on the back of the letter, which was never sent. It is undated but thought to be from c.1562, *Scritti ...*, p. 193n1.

This false opposition is easily done away with, because you can understand that before I would make this treatise known, I myself maintained that life for many decades, and we learn that others before me have maintained it, and now the many who have read my treatise maintain it. They believe that man should disdain the senses, which are proper to animals and contrary to reason, the virtue proper to man – and that he should want to live the life of a man as he truly can, by maintaining continence; and because maintaining continence and a sober life is not impossible but easy to do. Such a life consists of only two orders of the mouth: one, not to eat foods contrary to his stomach – there being many kinds of good foods that do not harm him – nor to drink wine contrary to that [stomach]; two, to eat good food and drink good wine, which should be eaten and drunk according to what the stomach of that man can easily digest. With these two orders we maintain a sober life. And when a man has reached the age of thirty-five or forty-five or fifty-five years, he also knows from past experience which foods and wines are good for his stomach and in which quantities, and by maintaining these two orders he maintains a sober life; which conserves man up to the said time, even if born with a poor complexion, as was I. And yet by virtue of Lady Continence, I have reached the age of ninety years in the best of health,[51] prosperous and content, and I will reach one hundred because at the age of forty years I fell in love with that beautiful Lady, and I have always embraced her day and night, and will always do so as she will me.

O how kind hearted a Lady she is and how her love benefits me! Nor is there another method or way to arrive to that end in good health, because whoever tries to reach it on the strength of a good complexion cannot reach it in good health, as it is the opinion of all who write and say that as a man reaches the age of eighty years he enters an age full of displeasure and pain, and now we see that this is so. But because there are many *sensuali,* the enemies of reason, who, without basis, say they hope to reach [their end] with their usual none sober life, since others have already done so; yet, they do not see they are following pure error. Indeed, this is the opinion of the wise: that it cannot be reached without the above contrary effects, because, as in Nature, it is not possible to reach such an end in good health based on a beautiful and strong complexion if they are not living a sober life, as we now know. And because those *sensuali,* in order to excuse themselves, say they have seen others who have reached that age, they are incapable of seeing

---

51 Cornaro is probably seventy-eight or eighty years old in 1562.

that it is not so. As it is common for a man, once he reaches the age of
seventy years – in order to make the old seem prosperous – to say that
he is eighty; just as it is common that once a man has arrived at sixty
he may say he is only fifty, in order to be younger. And so it is almost
certain that whoever says he is eighty years old may only be seventy; and
besides, this can easily be believed by others. For even if he is not [that
age] he might as well be, because to the young, whoever is forty seems
old, and after seeing him live over a period of time, he judges [that
person] to be older than his age. I am judged to be one hundred years
of age and many believe this, yet I am only ninety; and there is no one
here at my age in the city of Padua or in that of Venice who is not full
of infirmities, just as I am free of them. But let us suppose there is one,
who, by some miracle, may be healthy and has reached that age owing
to a good complexion: it does not ensure him of not becoming ill and
dying. And with this malice of thought he lives an unhappy life just as I,
having arrived by way of a sober life, live in happiness; because I am
certain neither to become ill nor to die if not from resolution when it
is my time. And this certainty allows me to live happily, being liberated
in old age of all the bitter fruit of any bestial sense and being full of the
sweetest fruit of blessed reason; so that now, neither passions nor perturbations or other fruit of the senses harm me, not even the thought
of death nor the pains afterward, because through reason I liberate
myself. I therefore enjoy, rather, I revel in this beautiful world, which
is the most beautiful for the one who knows how to make it beautiful,
by means of my Lady, and who enjoys this perfect age that, without any
doubt, is the most perfect. And as one who has lived through them all,
I can attest that it is an age filled with good times without contraries;
whereas at other ages those [good times] have many [contraries].

O what a happy age! And if I were to write about all of its entertain-
ments I would have to write a treatise, the way I have resolved to write
[this], because one of my pastimes is writing and composing for several
hours a day, to be helpful and for no other reason.

O what pleasure it is for me to write about things that for sixty years
now I have studied and practised, and which at this time and at this age
have matured, making it easy for me to write about! And I do so with
pleasure because my thinking is not filled with fumes rising from my
stomach and burdening my head. O how I enjoy this pastime and the
countless others of this happy age! So it is that every person must do
everything possible to attain them, and be free of harm from the bad

thought continually troubling a man as he sees himself grow old. And this will convert into good, because he would rather arrive at this happy age, to which you Lordship will arrive if you decide to fall in love with this Lady; and do not fear that her love should harm another that you love, because I warrant that she will benefit you. And you will live healthy, to the great pleasure of all your people and of many others in keeping the world beautiful.

XXVI

To the Magnificent and my Most Honourable Lordship Messer Alvise Cornaro

Padua al Santo [Via del Santo]

I believe, your Most Honourable Magnificent Lordship Alvise, that continence is beautiful, a rare virtue, and rightly is, as your Magnificence says so well, our beautiful and dear and sweet Lady. That this is true, though a person be strong or *liberale* [licentious], is seen by the fact that you cannot practise those [none sober] habits without harm or danger to the faculties or to your own person. But your sweet and gentle beloved has this advantage, which lets them be lauded and praised to the stars; nor, however, does she cease to safeguard our lives and faculties and to promise long and almost perpetual happiness. It is an act of charity that your Magnificence so lovingly with your words has motivated me, and made me eager for her beauty that she might also teach me the way, and by which means, I could hope to arrive at my desired end and be able to gather the various fruits of her friendship. To be sure, I have often felt how great is your courtesy and kindness; hence, there will never be a time that I do not admit how indebted I am to you. But if you were now to add also this – that you teach me to save and prolong my person for a long time in this world – when will I (though a hoarse and ailing swan) ever tire of singing and celebrating your praises all along these shores, and wherever else I may travel?

Truly, in regard to this, you have principally said that – just as for other benefits – through this precious and rare treasure of Continence, man serves his needs. Therefore, whether it is someone old or young, big or small, learned or wise, when he feels ill and wishes to be well, he need only think of returning to the diet and a sober life, which would help him live and be healthy once again. With this solution, if we were to keep practising it and keep it close at hand at all times, our bodies will be truly blessed and happy and all of us most fortunate; because we would never, or rarely, become ill and would stay in this life for as long as we would most want to stay. But I do not know why it is that as soon as we are better and up and out of bed, sadly we allow ourselves to be led by vain appetite; which leads to acquiring every one of our ills, and we do not see it. What the cause might be that makes us forget this most decent Lady, who so kindly embraces and preserves life, I still have not really been able to discover; and even if I knew, I could not hope she would help me unless your Magnificence, wise and experienced in this matter, were not to confirm this truth. Therefore, I appreciate the most beautiful gift of asparagus,[52] which at this time has come to me as undeniable proof of your infinite thoughtfulness and the love you have for me, and I ask of you the special favour of being so kind as to reveal this secret and make it known to me. For it truly is that if on earth one man can pride himself in knowing this, you are the one who should know it, since continuously and over the length of fifty years, as you say, you have always led that commendable life. Hence, it is not so much in some other person as much as in you alone that I place my faith in this matter. And it makes me think that, just as one should not simply believe in the medicine of a person who makes his profession [as a physician] out of that art – but who, nonetheless, does not know how to cure the infirm – so it is by my faith in your work that, not only by its words but by its very results, has shown how much its precepts do benefit and that it is the path to a healthy life. Once you have done this what other major good could you possibly desire? And so it will silence your detractors, who, if with good reason they believe that one Herodikos of Selymbria,[53] spending all his time in search of longevity and health – but did not cure souls nor nations nor friends nor had any honours – should be reprimanded, what can they then say about the person of your Magnificence, who has always strived to live a long life in good health, has always assisted his homeland and his nation and his family, discovering a wonderful invention for the reclamation and preservation of Venice's lagoon, and with his many numerous beautiful works – done by his own hand and ingenuity – has been able to make known the way and means

---

52 Asparagus is a diuretic and helpful as an "antilithic, those that break up kidney stones and purge the gravel from the bladder," apparently an ailment with a "painfully frequent occurrence in the Renaissance," K. Albala, *Eating Right …*, p. 100.
53 Herodikos of Selymbria (fifth century BCE), considered a Sophist, was a Thracian (Bulgarian) physician – teacher to Hippocrates (460–c.377 BCE) – and mentioned by Plato. He was also known as the "father of sports medicine."

of safeguarding our life for a long time from death's grip? But to this, Magnificence, you could say that classical philosophers and that rare book of yours – in the possession of all men – is that which teaches the ways and means to live a long life in good health, and to avoid illness. But it must be said that although those divine pages of your Magnificence, and the books by Plato, Aristotle, and Xenophon, teach how we may live soberly and to use continence, this does not, however, ensure that owing to these many precepts the world will not continue to live in a dissolute way and will not heed your ways. Thus, in addition to that most wise guidance, all of which I remember having read, I would like shown to me how I can unreservedly be rid of these godless tyrants that torment me, and thus be able to place myself safely in the embrace of this caring and rare Lady, so powerful a friend to your Magnificence that – out from the shadow of this age of ninety years – she has the power to let you live, and allows you more than ever to delight in and be amused by youthful thoughts. And here I conclude, praying to God from my heart that, if possible, He add to your joy and happiness and life and sweet thoughts.

5 May 1563.

Most beholden servant to your Magnificence,
Bartolamio Zacco[54]

---

54 Bartolameo (Bartolamio) Zacco (1522–1585), a very good friend of Speroni, was an acclaimed Paduan poet, and author of *Storia di Padova*.

Letter from Giacomo Alvise[55]

I believe that your Magnificence will not be displeased to learn about the condition of our exceptional old man, who is truly a marvel to behold though his life continues to weaken; nonetheless, he never ceases to give advice or practical suggestions and is so steadfast and firm in his disregard of death, one cannot in any way tell that he might need help during his usual activities. Though his tongue is quite swollen, his brain works and he remembers so much that it is astonishing; his thinking constantly seeks something new to benefit the world, as he did this evening when, having imagined a beautiful way to make a *carro*, as a way for transitioning at the Lizza Fusina,[56] he immediately called a servant and had him write it down, then this morning he sent for a sculptor and had him make a model in his presence. He is conducting other similar activities and continuously describes them, and so, this miracle, which in him finds more activities to do in the same amount of time that others only waste.

---

55 Cornaro's grandson. The addressee is unknown. It may be Cornaro's longtime, very close friend, Bishop Cornelio Musso, to whom he dedicated his *Vita sobria* in Tomitano's letter to Musso (*Sober ...*, p. 72).

56 The c*arro*, or transporter system, was an "ingenious" means of transitioning boats between the freshwater (Brenta River) and the seawater (Venice lagoon) and back. Although it was decreed in 1561 to replace them with a series of locks, the system remained in use until 1614–1615. It was even noted by Montaigne in 1580 as cited in the *Itinerario di Marin Sanuto* [Sanudo] ..., (1847), pp. ix–x, in note 11 by Rawdon Brown. And see for example, Violet M. Jeffery, "Shakespeare's Venice," in *Modern Language Review* 27, no. 1 (1932): pp. 24–35.

Fusina, at the mouth of the Brenta River, was an embankment located south of Venice.

If I were to write about the many other things, I would not finish today.
But I only wanted to advise you of these few things, my knowing that
since your Magnificence finds him worthy of your love then it should
also please you to have news of him during these his final days of life.
There remains only to tell you that he is also similarly composed in his
heart [*animo*] with God, and we plainly see that he loves Him out of
love, and does not fear Him out of fear, thus we must hope every good
for his soul.

For now I will say no more if not that to see him and to hear him,
since he brings us such pleasure and amazement, and seeing that we
will lose a man so full of goodness and other rare qualities brings us
pain and endless sorrow. But since it so pleases Him Who reigns over all
things, we must be content with His Will reminding us that we are born
to die, and he who dies well attains in this world and the next, immortality and a better life. And with this, I kiss your hand.

Padua, end of April 1566.[57]

From the friend of Your Illustrious Magnificence
[Signore Giacomo Luigi Cornaro Piscopia]

---

57 Cornaro died shortly after this letter was written. The date conventionally given as the
   day he died is 8 May 1566; but that date instead may have been the day of his funeral.
   See "Intro.," pp. 42–3.

How to Attain Immortality Living
One Hundred Years,
or, The Fortune of the *Vita Sobria* in the
Anglo-Saxon World*◊

Marisa Milani

It was during 1763 when Mr. Thomas Wood, resident of the village Billeri-cary in the County of Essex, miller by profession, big eater and big beer drinker, began to grow noticeably fat. By forty years of age, he was very fat and at forty-four he had begun to feel the first disturbances brought on by his bulging obesity: "he first began to be disturbed in his sleep, and to complain of the heart-burn, of frequent sickness at his stomach, pains in the bowels, head ache, and vertigo. He was sometimes costive, at other times the opposite extreme; had almost a constant thirst, a great lowness of spirit, violent rheumatism, and frequent attacks of the gout. He had likewise two epileptic fits. But the symptom, which appeared to him to be the most formidable, was a sense of suffocation, which often came to him, particularly after his meals." He went on like this for some months, indulging in fatty meats, which he ate three times a day, as well as large quantities of butter and cheese, not to mention the strong ale that he gulped down in staggering amounts. If he had continued on like that, he

---

* [Milani's essay – in Italian, "Come raggiungere l'immortalità vivendo cent'anni, ovvero La fortuna della 'Vita Sobria' nel mondo anglosassone," in *Cultura Neolatina* 40, nos. 4, 5, 6 (Modena: S.T.E.M.- Mucchi, 1980), pp. 333–56 – is translated into English for the first time here in the Da Ponte edition.

    NB: A citation in English without square brackets is transcribed as cited by Milani in the original essay.

    Information in English regarding titles and publications – as found in the notes to "Immortality ...," – was transcribed as per Milani's original citations; that is, odd spellings are common to the times they were written. *Citations rendered into English by this translator are enclosed in single square brackets.*]

◊ [A note within single square brackets [] – accompanied by an asterisk *, or diamond – was inserted by this translator.]

certainly would not have lived for long, but fortunately for him the Reverend Mr. Powley, "a worthy clergyman in the neighbourhood," evidently concerned about the health and not just the souls of his faithful, seeing the miller ever fatter and in a bad way, one day advised him to go on a diet, recommending a book suitable to that end – *The Life of Cornaro* – "as a book likely to suggest to him a salutary course of living." Mr. Wood obtains the book, reads it, and becomes so enthused he immediately begins a strict diet, which in a few years restores him to perfect health in body and spirit. There are reliable witnesses who signed a declaration to this effect on 30 January 1770. Among them was Mr. Benjamin Pugh, "Physician at Chelsford," who had often visited the miller, measuring his pulse and examining his urine: "He makes everyday," – the doctor certifies – "about a pint and half of urine, which is a full amber colour. It had scarce varied, either in quantity or apparence [*sic*], ever since he left off drinking."

If from a medical point of view the case of Mr. Wood appears extraordinary and worthy of note (and accepted as such in *Medical Transactions*), it is even more extraordinary for one who takes an interest not in diets but in the fate of a text. The miraculous book recommended by the English physician was indeed none other than the *Trattato de la vita sobria* [Treatise on the sober life] by Alvise Cornaro, whose [first] discourse was issued in Padua by the publisher Perchacino [*sic*] in 1558, rapidly followed by another three in 1561, 1563, and 1565, respectively.

Historical European medical and paramedical culture is abound with treatises and dietary advice, from that of Michele Savonarola dedicated to Borso d'Este around the middle of the Quattrocento, to modern studies, but none have survived beyond a few decades. Moreover, they limit their advice to one of indicating models of alimentation, none advise a radical change of life or habit as does that of Cornaro, who presents himself to the reader as the prime example and proof of the authenticity of his own claims. Cornaro is the only one to demonstrate through his own longevity the healthiness of his method: how do we not believe someone, practically a centenarian, who extols the model for living – which he himself has followed for well over fifty years – as the sure means not only for avoiding illness and for attaining one's oldest age but for actually attaining a serene death absent of pain?

There is no doubt that the fate of his treatise lies in this easy explanation. Lending credence to this, is an English edition from 1935 in which George Cooke, author of the introduction, expresses himself as follows:

There have been many writers of books about food and health; and many people have lived to be a hundred. But, as far as I know, Luigi Cornaro is the only man (with the possible exception of Hippocrates ...) who has adopted a special system of eating, has written various treatises about it, and has lived for a hundred years. Or very nearly a hundred. Cornaro's exact age at the time of his death is not quite certain but he must have been over ninety-eight.

As such, his works have a peculiar importance. Many books have been written on the subject of longevity and many suggestions have been put forward by which a long life could be attained and death could be warded off. But these theories have not been successful in actual practice and their authors have, as a rule, lived no longer than other men.[1]

And so proceeding, he speaks on the diet of Cornaro:

> Now in many respects this system is absolutely opposed to the conclusions of our modern doctor and dieticians. But, while their theories are the result of laboratory work and experiments on animals, Cornaro's diet was based on a completely successful experiment on himself (...). Of course he is only one case, and what suited him may not suit everybody, as he says himself. But I suggest that his principles deserve a close and imprejudiced examination, We may yet discover that he knew more about diet than our modern scientific authorities. (9)*

The studies by Emilio Menegazzo have shown Cornaro to be an accomplished liar in regard to his own age and that he does not die at the cusp of one hundred years, as he would have you believe, but at "only" eighty-two.[2] An enviable end for anyone but not for the one who had decided that, since Nature was not averse to his arriving at 120 years, a sober life would have allowed him to reach it, or at least to touch upon one

---

1 *How to Live for a Hundred Years and Avoid Disease.* A Treatise by Luigi Cornaro the Sixteenth Century Italian Centenarian. Translated by George Herbert with an Introduction by George Cooke Comparing Cornaro's System with Modern Theories of Diet (Oxford: The Alden Press, 1935), p. 7.

* [Parenthetical numbers inserted here in this essay are page references to works listed only within Milani's footnotes. They do not refer to pages in the Da Ponte edition (*Sober ...,*).]

2 Emilio Menegazzo, "Altre osservazioni intorno alla vita e all'ambiente del Ruzante e di Alvise Cornaro," *Italia Medioevale e Umansitica* 9 (1966): pp. 229–62.

hundred; and his goal seemed to be near, given that – when he claimed
this in Discourse IV – he said he was 95 years old. Half a decade before,
in a letter to the Great Commander of Cyprus in 1551, he maintained
with extreme confidence:

> [...think *Signore* ...I am more than healthy, and more than prosperous, and
> for that very reason I conclude, that I cannot die owing to an illness that
> may befall me, but only out of resolution, caused only by my very old age,
> but not before one hundred, or more, years].[3]

With such claims often repeated in his writings it is understandable that,
knowing his strength would not endure over so long a time, he would
have resorted to a little trickery in progressively increasing his years so as
to make it seem that, if not actually, he was at least nudging the end he
had predetermined. And that he was to succeed in this is demonstrated by
the fact that none of those who knew him, not even his relatives or most
intimate friends, had raised any doubts, rather, through their testimonials
they all reinforced the fame of the centenarian. One should add that
Cornaro did not act out of some silly peculiarity of old age, nor was it an
innocent lie, but the conscious act of a man who his entire life never admitted
to being wrong, and fought until the end with all his might against
anyone who did not accept his theories or disagreed with him. Evidence
of this is in his writings on the reclamation of the lagoon, his conflicts with
Sabbadino and the Venetian Signory, the quarrel with Cardinal Pisani, and
the civil but ongoing polemics with Speroni in regard to sober living. Not
to mention how he succeeded in accomplishing for his descendants the
much hoped for title of nobility by having his only daughter marry the
noble, though not wealthy, Giovanni Cornaro Piscopia, so compliant that
he accepts that his firstborn – who, according to tradition, would take the
name of the paternal grandfather – instead takes the name of his father-
in-law's deceased brother. It is a detail of little account, if you like, but one
that nevertheless shows Cornaro's authority as the grand *pater familias*.

If no one from the Cornaro circle manifested doubts, readers of the
Vita sobria had even less, and Alvise Cornaro passed into the medical
and paramedical literature of the past four centuries as the supreme

---

3 From the Cod[ex] Lat[ino]. 6251 at the National Library of Vienna, f. 78r. The letter,
   fols. 77r–82r, is a copy with corrections and additions by the same hand. The change
   of dates is interesting: *Di Padova adi. 23. Zenaro 1551* becomes *Di Pad.a alli ... Febraro*
   [15]51.

and irrefutable proof of health and longevity. Some uncertainty – soon dispelled – arose, if at all, in regard to the quantity of food and drink that he was said to take: the famous 12 *'alla sotile'* [short] ounces of food and the 14 of wine.[4] Cardano, for example, in one of his dialogues, says that it is unclear from the context if the quantity refers to a single meal or covers the daily diet,[5] but in his major work, the *De Sanitate Tuenda* [on care of health], he proposes Cornaro as an example of those sickly persons who *dum caute vivant, diutius vivunt* [living cautiously, live longer].[6] In

---

4 "(…) onde io per non parer ostinato e più medico di essi medici et sopra tutto per compiacer i miei che questo molto desideravano giudicando essi che tale augumento mi havesse a conservar la vita contentai di acrescer il cibo ma in due oncie sole più, che sì come prima tra pane un rosso d'uovo carne, et minestra mangiava tanto ch'in tutto pesasse oncie dodici alla sotile così poi lo crescei a oncie quatordici, et sì come prima beveva oncie quatordeci de vino così poi crescei alle sedici" (I, 175a). Following this, with minimal changes graphically, is the text from the Paolo Meietto edition (Padua, 1591), transcribed in the Codex Vienna, but for the benefit of the reader, the pages of the Fiocco edition are given (G[iuseppe] Fiocco, *Alvise Cornaro, il suo tempo e le sue opere* (Vicenza, 1965). Discourse I is revised in the 1558 edition.

5 We cite the passage that in the French version accompanies the text by Cornaro, and was passed on in later English translations: "Il semble donc que Cornaro ait voulu nous ôter la conoissance parfaite de son régime, & se contenter de nous apprendre qu'il en avoit trouvé un merveilleux, puisqu'il ne nous a point marqué s'il prenoit cette quantité une ou deux fois par jour, ni même s'il changeoit d'alimens, & qu'il a parlé sur ce sujet d'une manière encore plus obscure qu'Hypocrate. Cependant on doit conjecturer qu'il ne prenoit cette quantité de nourture qu'une fois par jour, & qu'il y apportoit quelque variété, puisque s'il en prenoit quelque fois davantage, il régloit ce qui excédoit sur le poids d'un raisin ou d'une figue. Il y a encore lieu de s'étonner que sa boisson excédât ses alimens solides, d'autant plus que ce qu'il mangeoit n'étoit pas également nourrissant, puisqu'il y avoit des jaunes d'oeufs & de la viande. En vérité, il me paroît plutôt parler en Philosophe qu'en Médecin" (*Dialogue de Cardan, Entre un Philosophe, un Citoyen & un Hermite, sur la manière de prolonger la vie, & de conserver la santé*). From the *Liber secundus* del *Theonoston. Seu De Vita Producenda, atque incolumitate corporis conservanda,* in Hieronymi Cardani Mediolanensis Philosophi ac Medici celeberrimi *Operum* Tomus secundus; quo continentur *Moralia quaedam et Physica* (Lugduni, M.DC.LXIII), pp. 372–402 (p. 376a).

6 Hieronymi Cardani Mediolamensis, Ciuisq. Bononiensis, Medici Clarissimi *Opus nouum cunctis de SANITATE TVENDA, ac vita producenda studiosis apprime necessarium: in quatuor libros digestum.* A Rodulpho Sylvestro Bononiensi Medico, recens in lucem editum. Ad Gregorium XIII. Pont. Max. (Romae, Anno MDLXXX).

   Here are the two passages regarding Cornaro: "Secunda fuit ratio Aloysij Cornarij, qui uentriculo laborans, cum circa annum aetatis XXXVI. pro deplorato haberetur, sibi rationem uitae pondere pręscripsit cibi duodecim vnciarum in dies, potus quatuordecim, nec ab illa discedens magnam consecutus est foelicitatem, sanus corpore, victis litibus, quibus ditatus est, suscepto filio, & ex eo octo nepotibus, cum esset nobilis Venetus, ac prudens, magnum attulit temperantiae suae exemplum, & emolumentum. Quin

1702, in his response to a successful French translation of the *Vita sobria*, nothing less than an *Anti-Cornaro* emerges.[7]

Among his contemporaries, one of those less than convinced to follow his "loving exhortation" was Sperone Speroni, who responds thus to a letter by Cornaro:

> To be sure, I believe many of these things to be true, and I am certain that just as a crippled hand is not a hand because it cannot operate otherwise, so too the sober life is not life but half-death, because it does not operate as much as or in the way a man should operate. And I believe that to die from resolution, which your Magnificence glorifies, is the worst manner of death possible for a man, because it is to die from starvation (…) Moreover, to die from resolution is troublesome not just for the one who dies in this way, but also for the one who sees him die in this way (…).There would then be the danger that in seeing a man die of starvation out of resolution, (…) that he be buried before having finished, or that he be strangled out of compassion. (…) Your Magnificence will say that I do well to defend disorder, living disordered [as I do], which my leg can attest. My response is that it is enough for me living more soberly than a man in Rome, and without need of a back brace for a man of my age; and may God grant that in me the pain that should go to my head alone should all go to my legs. (…) I am almost sixty-two years of age, and Your Magnificence began to regulate his life at the age of forty. Habit is a great thing, and just as whoever was to impose disorder on you now would kill you, so too whoever was to impose order on me now would kill me. (…) Writing after meals, Your Magnificence must remember, is healthy for you or at least does not harm you, but for me it would be harmful; therefore you do it, and I do not. On this, which is eminently clear, I will say nothing more and conclude that many philosophers

---

excussus e carpento etiã rursus prẹter spem medicodum euasit. Hoc exemplum sequuti sunt non pauci. Dominicus Saulus, Gabriel Panigarola, ac Leonicenus, qui omnes morbis inexpugnabilibus laborãtes ad longam senectam peruenere, & incolumi etiam corpore: Cornarius ad XCVII (… .)" (*liber quartus*, 283 B). "Alij cum saepe aegrotent, ad senectam perueniunt: horum igitur causam prius discere expedit, nam ea non intellecta, neque licebit omnino propositum assequi. Tres igitur causae sunt, quibus alterna illa vicissitudo accidit. Prima est confidentia in his qui sani degũt, dum perlicita omnia, & illicita ruunt: sibique mortem approperant, contra, aegri dum caute uiuant, diutius uiuunt, velut de Aloysio Cornario saepe dictum est" (*ibid.*, 285 DE).

The Meietto edition of the *Vita sobria* will also be dedicated to Gregory XIII.

7 *L'Anti-Cornaro, ou Remarques critiques sur le Traité de la Vie Sobre de Louis Cornaro* (Paris, 1702).

and a great many saints died young, who, on the other hand, did not have to live less than soberly, while many wicked and ignorant carnal persons arrived at one hundred years, to where – so God may grant me the happiness of my blood [family] and my friends – I would not like to arrive dying the way they do. Therefore, I will not kill myself nor will I do anything where nourishment would operate to kill me, but I will live far removed from this desire, and from this cure [of a sober life].[8]

Much more perfunctory is the judgment of Aretino:

> (…) rispondo a chi dice, che nel seguire de gli appetiti si accelera la morte, che l'huomo tanto si prolunga la vita, quanto adempisce i suoi desideri, et ciò dico io, e non Plato.[9]

> (…) my response to whoever says that in following your appetites you hasten death, is that man prolongs his life for as long as he can fulfill his desires, and that is what I say, not Plato.

The criticisms and dismissals by such distinguished men did not at all tarnish the fame that Cornaro went on to claim and which, in 1580, we have seen consolidated in the treatise of one of the most authoritative physicians of the time, Cardano. Little more than twenty years had passed since the 1558 appearance of [Cornaro's] first discourse, which was followed in 1561 by the second (*Compendio breve della Vita Sobria* [brief Compendium of the sober life]), still with the Paduan printer Perchacino; accordingly his *Lettera al Barbaro* [Letter to B.] in 1563 and *Amorevole Essortatione* [*Loving Exhortation*] in 1565 were also printed with the same publisher. The complete edition of his four discourses will appear only in 1591, edited by Evangelista Oriente for the printer Meietto in Padua – in which, however, the *Exhortation* precedes the *Letter* – with the title of, *Discorsi della vita sobria del Sr. Luigi Cornaro*.

The work was read by the [Flemish] Jesuit, Leendert Leys, better known by his Latin name Leonardus Lessius, whose enthusiasm brought him to the point of applying the teachings of Cornaro on himself, and of

---

8 From Rome, 22 February 1562. The text conforms to the Codex Vienna, fols. 33r–36v. Cf. S. Speroni, *Opere* (Venice, 1740), III, p. 414ff.

9 Cornaro is not named, but it appears that, given the topic under discussion, it may very well be about him. It is the letter to Speroni from Venice dated December 1547. Pietro Aretino, *Lettere*, I. IV (Paris, 1608), pp. 130–1.

writing in the wake of his master a treatise in Latin on the same theme, to which he places in an appendix a [Latin] translation of Cornaro's first discourse.[10] In the dedicatory letter to the Magnificent Reverend Father Rumoldo, he justifies the translation of Cornaro thus:

> Adiunxi Tractatum cuiusdam Veneti, viri sanè pręclari, & acris iudicij, Ludovici Cornari, eódem pertinentem: qui, longa experientia, quanta sit Sobrietatis, didicit, eamque scripto suo egregiè cõmendat. (3r)

> [I have added a treatise by a man from the Veneto, a truly remarkable man, and of penetrating judgment, Ludovico Cornaro, to whom [the treatise] belongs, and who, through lengthy experience, came to know the high value of sobriety and in his letter praised it brilliantly.]*

In addition, explaining how he came to know about Cornaro's works:

> Haec cogitanti [[salute e vecchiaia]] exibitus est à viro illustri libellus quidam de Vita Sobria, Italico sermone conscriptus, auctore D. Ludouico Cornaro Veneto, magni ingenij viro, honorato, opulento, & coniugij vinculis adstricto, in quo mirificè haec ratio commendatur omnibus, & multâ certâque experientiâ comprobatur. Valdè recreatus fui libelli huius lectione, planeq. dignum iudicaui, quem in Latinum sermonem translatum omnibus facerem communem: praemisso hoc meo tractatu exegetico. (3–4)

> [In consideration of these things [[health and old age]] is a booklet presented by an illustrious man on the sober life, written in the Italian language by the Venetian author Dom Ludovico Cornaro – a man of great innate quality, respected, affluent, and committed to the bond of marriage – in which, in a wonderful way, this order is recommended to everyone and is demonstrated by ample and certain experience. I was greatly invigorated after reading this booklet, and I judged it utterly worthy, which, translated into Latin, I made accessible to all: having placed it ahead of my exegetic treatise.]

---

10 *Hygiasticon seu Vera Ratio Valetudinis Bonae et Vitae unà cum Sensuum, Iudicii, & Memoriae integritate ad extremam senectutem cõseruandae: Auctore* Leonard Lessio, *Societatis Iesu Theologo. Subiungitur Tractatus* Lvdovici Cornari *Veneti, eódem pertinens, ex Italico in Latinum sermonem ab ipso* Lessio *translatus.* (*Antuerpiae,* Ex Officina Platiniana, Apud Viduam & Filios Io. Moreti. M.DC.XIII).

    On pages 74ff: Lvdovici Cornari Veneti *Tractatus de Vitae Sobriae Commodis. L'editio secunda,* in fact a reprint, is dated M.DC.XIV.

* [My thanks to Da Ponte series editor, Prof Massimo Ciavolella, for his invaluable assistance with translating the Latin.]

Almost fifty years after the death of Cornaro, therefore, his treatise continues to be read and discussed, at least by the *illustres viri* [illustrious men] familiar with Italian, and with the Lessius translation [in Latin], the fame of Cornaro decisively crosses borders to spread throughout Europe. His success is immediate, and it is enhanced by the discussions and debates that the work incites. Once again, it is above all the diet that is discussed, on the matter of the 12 and 14 ounces. We hear it echo in a curious appendix placed by the unknown owner of the 1558 Venetian edition now in the Bodleian Library at Oxford.[11] On the two blank pages in the back, precisely written in careful imitation of the book's printed characters, are these letter excerpts:

The Lord Duke of Urbino, in the letter written the 2nd of October 1613 to the Count of Bruay, says:

Here, at other times, consideration was made on that rule for living which Cornaro was following, and it was believed that where he speaks of twelve ounces of food and fourteen of drink he means, not for the day, but at one meal and it appears that he still has that egg yolk, which cannot be divided up, so that it would not be so strict a thing as it appears on the face of it, although to place oneself under so exact an order seems that there may be some harm done or danger if it were to be altered in any way, as he tells about what happened to him for having increased his food by only two ounces and likewise his drink.

Father Lessius in an epistle from Leuven dated the first of September in the year 1613 to the Count of Bruay.

Cum ego duodecim uncias cibi constituo loquor de pane et obsonijs non de panatella uel menestra, loquor aquae uel uini qui ibi ad mensuram potus pertinet; panis commixtus ad mensuram cibi, ut si sint quatuor unciae aquae uel uini in panatella tanto minus sumendum in potu et detrahendum ex quatuordecim uncijs potui assignatis. Cornaro tumetiamsi panatella computaretur in cibis duodecim unciae satis erant, mihi duodecim unciae cibi etiam sunt nimium, in potu sufficiunt nouem uel decem, quid faciēdum illis qui exactam illam rationem dietae seruare nequeunt, dixi in tractatu num° 27°. An uaria dietae mensura uarijs aetatibus conueniat, non est dubitandū: nemini tum maiorest conueniens, quā quae apté a stomacho confici queat, ita ut nulla relinquatur cruditas: idex regulis traditis adhibita experientia facile potest deprehendi: ualde tamē ab omnibus medicis improbatur magna ciborum

---

11 *Trattato de la Vita Sobria del Magnifico M. Luigi Cornaro Nobile Vinitiano.* In Venice, at San Luca al segno del Diamante, n.d. (but 1558). The shelf mark is *Holk,* fol. 59.

uarietas et exquisitus apparatus condiendorum, quo fit ut cibi ita alterentur ut nescias sitne caro an piscis, uelut an pulpa ceruis, uitulina an caprina.

[Since I prepare twelve ounces of food, I speak of bread and side-dishes not of panatella or soup, I speak of water or wine, which here relate to the amount for drinking, to the right amount of bread combined with foods; so that, if there are four ounces of water or wine in the panatella, the same amount must be taken from drinking, and must be subtracted from the fourteen ounces assigned to drink. Therefore, even if for Cornaro the panatella is thought to be enough food in the amount of twelve ounces, for me twelve ounces of food is too much, and drinking nine or ten [ounces] is sufficient, which should be done by those unable to adhere to so exact a system of diet, as I stated in treatise number XXVII. And one should not doubt whether a different quantity of diet is appropriate at different ages: what is appropriate is what can be consumed well by the stomach, so that no excess may remain: its applied practice can easily be understood from the rules handed down. However, all physicians strongly condemn [too] great a variety of foods and the delectable supply of savouries, which result in foods that alter in such a way that you would not know if it is meat or fish, or the flesh of deer, or calf or goat.]

Pater Lessius in margine epistolae suae ad Comitem de Bruay Iouanio decimal quinta mensis May 1614.

Mitto exemplar secundę editionis de sanitate tuenda ubi paucula addita exmonitione E. V. ut uidere est numero decimo-quinto: scribitur Roma ab Ill.mis Cardinalibus lectitari.

[Father Lessius in the margin of his epistle to Count of Bruay of Leuven on 15 of May 1614.

I am sending a copy of the second edition of the *De Sanitate Tuenda*, in which very few of the admonitions from E.V. are added, as seen in number XV: it is written that in Rome it was eagerly read by the Most Illustrious Cardinals.]

The presence of a single addressee for the letters makes us think that the owner of the book could very well be the Count of Bruay, who, enthused after reading the Lessius translation, may have wanted to deepen his knowledge, or dispel his own doubts, by requesting a reply from the translator and keen supporter of Cornaro on the one hand, and [a reply] from the Duke of Urbino, who appears to head up an array of sceptics on the other. This, all in the quick turnover of the mail, if one considers that the *Hygiasticon* obtains the *Summa Privilegii* of the Archdukes of Austria on 25 June 1613 and the Lessius letter follows by only two months, while that of the duke by three. It really does seem that with its first appearance the work of Cornaro – more than that of its translator – had raised a small tempest within the cultured circles of Europe. Seeming to confirm this is the second piece by Lessius, who, to settle the question that arose between the two contenders, sends the count a copy of Cardano in which, as we know, contrary to his dialogue, he gives credit to what Cornaro had said.

But if Latin was the only means to reach a European intellectual circle, it was also an impassable obstacle for the great numbers of those who did not know it, and the need was soon felt that the golden rules of life set out by Lessius and Cornaro should be made widely available. It is the reason why the first translations began to appear – beginning with the manuscripts but soon after in print – which will be republished up to the present time. The first known published translation is the English one of 1634, followed by the one in French by Sébastien Hardy in 1646, and a German one in 1653, and so forth. We will concern ourselves here only with the English translations, which, for their numbers, reworkings, revivals, and reprintings – in uninterrupted succession for more than three centuries – offer a material as rich as it is intricate.[12]

The first translations of the treatise by Lessius and the one by Cornaro – the former the work of the same publisher who signs himself only with the initials T.S., the latter the work of the famous and venerated George Herbert – turn up at Cambridge in 1634.[13] It is the same T.S. who explains to the reader (*To the Reader. The Preface of the Publisher of the ensuing Treatises*: 4v–7r) the presence of two translations:

---

12 The article by William E. A. Axon, "Cornaro in English," in *The Library*, N.S. II (1901), pp. 120–9, is so full of errors and inaccuracies as to often go astray.

13 *Hygiasticon: or The right course of preserving Life and Health unto extream old Age: Together with foundnesse and integritie of the Senses, Judgement and Memorie*. Written in Latine by *Leonard Lessius*, And now done into English. (Printed by Roger Daniel, printer to the Universitie of Cambridge, 1634). Following the text is Cornaro's treatise (*A Treatise of Temperance and Sobrietie*. Written by *Lud. Cornarus*. Translated into English by Mr. *George Herbert*) with a new enumeration that also includes a brief discourse, not mentioned in the titles (*A discourse translated out of Italian*), attributed by Axon to Ortensio Lando (Axon, p. 124).

Master *George Herbert* of blessed memorie, having at the request of a Noble Personage translated it into English, sent a copie thereof, not many
moneths before his death, unto some friends of his, who a good while before had given an attempt of regulating themselves in matter of *Diet*: Which,
although it was after a very imperfect manner, in regard of that exact course
therein prescribed; yet was of great advantage to them, inasmuch as they
were enabled, through the good preparation that they had thus made, to go
immediately to the practise of that pattern, which *Cornarus* hath set them,
and so have reaped the benefit thereof, in a larger and eminenter manner
then could otherwise possibly have been imagined in so short a space.

    Not so long after, *Lessius* his book, by happie chance, or, to speak better,
by gracious providence of the *Author of Health* and all other good things,
came to their hands: Whereby receiving much instruction and confirmation, they requested from me the Translation of it into English. Whereupon
hath ensued what you shall now receive. (4v–5r)

According to Axon (122–3) the noble friend who made the request
must have belonged to the circle of the famous Protestant Nunnery,
founded circa 1630 by Nicholas Ferrar at Little Gidding. Yet, nothing was
more likely, given the ascetic life conducted within the convent. The translation of Cornaro, therefore, circulated in manuscript form, and it was
only upon request that the *Hygiasticon* was also printed. We might ask the
question as to why Cornaro was preferred over the Jesuit and perhaps the
explanation lies in a practical reason: the manuscript of Cornaro's treatise
– remember, only the first discourse [1558] was given – was better suited
to being passed around, which, as a manual of dietary norms and advice,
a small community was able to apply. Herbert knew the Lessius text very
well, if for no other reason than it was the Latin translation from which he
derived his own. Up to then, no one had doubted that Herbert's translation might not have been based on the original, whether it was because it
was simply assumed, (although on a closer look, there is the fact that in
the titles the *Hygiasticon* is specified "Written in Latin (…) and now done
into English," and for the third text it speaks of "A discourse translated out
of Italian," while for that of Herbert, not speaking of it can be significant),
or whether it was because the same Herbert had resorted to a little subter-
fuge: the passage where Cornaro cites the two proverbs on food:

(…) allegava quei due proverbij naturali, et verissimi: l' uno è che chi vuol
mangiar assai bisogna che mangi poco (…) l'altro che giova più quel cibo che
si resta di mangiare quando si ha ben mangiato che non giova quello che già
si ha mangiato (…). (174a)

is translated as:

> To this agreed two Italian Proverbs, the one whereof was, *He that will eat much, let him eat little* (...) The other Proverb was, *The meat which remaineth, profits more than that which is eaten.* (18)

It is the exact version as in the text by Lessius:

> Huc pertinere duo prouerbia apud Italos vsitata. Alterum: *Qui multum vult comedere, comedat parum* (...). Alterum: *Plus iuuat cibus qui superest comedenti, quam qui ab illo comestus.* (86)

Except that Herbert refers to the two proverbs in a note, made to look like citations of the original but evidently fished from some Italian collection of the era:

> Mangierà più, chi manco mangia. Ed è contrario, Chi più mangia, manco mangia.
> Il senso è, Poco vive, chi troppo sparecchia.
> Fa più pro quel che si lascia sul' tondo, che quel' che si mette nel ventre.
>
> [He will eat more, who hardly eats. And the corollary is —Who eats more, hardly eats.
> The sense is – he lives less who too often cleans his plate.
> What we leave on our plate does more than what we put in our belly.]

In regard to the text – which can also be explained by remembering to whom it was sent – Herbert had few scruples about censoring anything that seemed to his faithful Protestant eye too papist, on which T.S. excuses him while refusing to use the same method because,

> Neither his [[Cornaro's]] old blinde zeal, nor the new and dangerous profession of *Lessius,* will (as we hope) breed any scandal or discredit to these present works of theirs, nor to the Imitatours of them, with any discreet and sincere Protestants. That they were both *Papists,* and the one of them a *Jesuite,* is no prejudice to the truth of what they write concerning *Temperance.* (5r–v)[14]

---

14 "To the Reader" is dated 7 December 1633.

Lessius had translated Cornaro's discourse by dividing it into 26 paragraphs, often preceded by an explanation of the theme to be discussed:
the original text is faithfully followed, with only two minimal omissions, a
brief explicative parenthesis, and the addition at the end of the last passage in the fourth discourse.[15] Herbert censors the entire introductory
part, and begins about halfway through ¶ 5:

> Having observed in my time many of my friends, of excellent wit and noble
> disposition, overthrown and undone by Intemperance; who, if they had
> lived would have been an ornament to the world, and a comfort to their
> friends: I thought fit to discover in a short Treatise (...) (1–2);

> cf. Lessius:

> Vidi ego multos ex meis amicis praestantissimi ingenij & nobilis naturae,
> florenti aetate abreptos ista peste intemperantiae, qui si viuerent, essent &
> mundo ornamento, & multis mortalibus solatio. Itaque ut tantis damnis oc-
> curam in posterum, statui hoc brevi discursu patefacere (...). (77)[16]

The translation proceeds without variation with respect to the Latin
until halfway through ¶ 19 and resumes at the beginning of ¶ 22 (from
"*Non è dubbio però ...*" 177b, to "*Ora perché alcuni uomini ...,*" 178a):
a censoring of the religious considerations that Cornaro expresses at this
point. In the final part, Herbert condenses into a few lines the paragraphs
23 to 26 (from "*Questi sono i sollazzi ...*" to the end, 180b s). Like Lessius,

---

15 Lessius omits the passage between parentheses in the text "(et perché la natura non
ci vieta (...) in tutto alla ragione)" (p. 172a); he avoids the repetitive redundancy of
the fragment "et già quattro anni (...) a sustentar una età vechia" (p. 174b) reducing it, with his characteristic succinctness to: "Quatuor iam anni sunt (accidit enim
cum 78 essem annorum) cum Medicorum consilio, & meorum importunitate assidua
inductus sum, ut aliquid mensurae consuetae adiicerem. Varias rationes adferebat:
senilem aetatem non posse tam modico cibo & potu sustentari" (pp. 85–6). Where
there is a parenthesis, it is added. At the end, he directly inserts with an indication in
the margin, "*Ex alio tractatu pag. 22 quem scripsit anna atatis* [*sic*] *XCV ad religioso,*" the
passage "*oh se questi si mettessero (...) questo per immense bontà,*" which is the ending of
Discourse IV (p. 190ab).

16 Cf. "Che ho io veduto morir de questa peste in fresca etade molti miei amici di belis-
simo inteletto, et di gentil natura, i quali se fossero vivi abbellirebono il mondo, Et
con mio gran contento sarebbono da me goduti, sì come con molto mio dolore di
loro son restato privo: onde per ovviar a tanto danno per l'avenir ho deliberato con
questo mio breve discorso far conoscere (...)". (pp. 171b–2a).

not even Herbert – or for that matter, any of the other translators – reveals the incongruity between the two ages that Cornaro attributes to himself in the text: the 81 years proclaimed at the beginning become 83 when he talks about the comedy he says he has written.

We find the translation by Herbert, always paired with the *Hygiasticon*, in a reprint of 1636 which is given as a third edition,[17] and again in 1678 in London in a different edition: in regard to the text, nothing is changed if not for some updating to the design and corrections according to the *errata* of the first edition.[18] The style of Herbert and the incompleteness of the text ensured that his version would be rebuffed in the following centuries; it will reappear partially changed and often summarized at Oxford in 1935 to serve as the basis for the medical-dietary considerations of one Mr. George Cook cited above.

At the dawn of the new century, in 1702, a new version is brought to English readers: this time not only is the treatise by Lessius eliminated but uniting with the first discourse are the three others as well, in addition to the letter from the Nun, the great-niece of Cornaro's, and the sayings and maxims on the subject.[19] The translator is W. Jones, who, in his *Preface*, thus declares with ill-concealed pride:

---

17 *Hygiasticon, etc.* The third Edition. (Printed by the Printers to the Universitie of Cambridge, 1636). The second edition is likely from 1635.

18 *The Temperate Man, or the Right Way of Preserving Life and Health, together, With Soundness of the Senses, Judgment, and Memory unto extream Old Age.* In Three Treatises. The First written by the Learned *Leonard Lessius.* The Second by *Lodowick Cornaro,* a Noble Gentleman of *Venice.* The third by a Famous Italian. Faithfully Englished. (London, Printed by J.R. for *John Starkey,* at the *Miter* in *Fleet Street,* near *Temple Bar,* 1678).

 Cornaro's title appears in continuation to Lessius (pp. 130–56): *A Treatise of Temperance an[d] Sobriety.* Written by Lud. Cornarus, Translated into English by Mr. George Herbert.

19 [* The "Nun's Letter" is not included in this Da Ponte edition. For a French source see the "Intro.," note 71, for an English source, see:] *Sure and Certain Methods of Attaining a Long and Healthful Life: with Means of Correcting a Bad Constitution, &c.* Written Originally in *Italian* by *Lewis Cornaro,* a Noble Venetian, when he was near an hundred Years of Age. And made *English* by *W. Jones,* A.B. (London, Printed for *Tho. Leigh,* and *Dan. Midwinter,* at the *Rose and Crown* in *St. Paul's Church-yard.* 1702).

 Chapter titles: I. *Of a Sober and Regular Life;* II. *The Method of Correcting a Bad Constitution;* III. *A Letter to Signior Barbaro, Patriarch of Aquileia; concerning the Method of enjoying a compleat Happiness in Old Age;* IV. *Of the Birth and Death of Man;* V. *Being a Letter from a Nun of Padua, the Grand-Daughter [sic] of Lewis Cornaro;* VI. *Authorities taken from the History of M. de Thou; and the Dialogues of Cardan concerning the Method of prolonging a Man's Life, and preserving his Health. Maxims to be observed for the prolonging of Life.*

The first Chapter [[of *A Sober and Regular Life*]]* was formerly publish'd in English in the small Tract of *Lessius* concerning Health, but so far mutilated, that it is not the same with the Original, and falls very much short of it. How it came to pass that it was thus lamely handed into the World, we shall not now enquire, but it may very fairly serve as a Justification for our New Version of that Discourse, especially since we have rendered the whole, and joyn'd three other Discourses, with other Matters relating thereto. It was thought proper to leave out some few things, which being writ by a Stanch *Roman* Catholick, seem'd to reflect upon the Protestant Religion; but hating this, you have the whole of *Cornaro's* Treatises, digested into so many distinct Chapters.

(…) our Reader (…) will thank *Cornaro* for the Original, and Us for the Version of it.[20]

Upon this Jones version an incredible fortune will smile: the second edition is from 1704, the third – with the translator unnamed and with a passage from the article by Addison that appeared in the *Spectator*, October 1711[21] – is released in 1722, the fourth, perhaps in 1727,[22] and the fifth, completely similar to the third, comes out in 1737. A full reprint of this last will return at a distance of more than a century later in

---

* [Inserted by Milani.]

20 The pages are not enumerated.

21 III, N. 195: "The most remarkable Instance of the Efficacy of Temperance towards the procuring of long Life, is what we meet with in a little Book publish'd by *Lewis Cornaro* the *Venetian*; which I the rather mention, because it is of undoubted Credit, as the late *Venetian* Ambassador, who was of the same Family, attested more than once in Conversation, when he resided in *England*. *Cornaro*, who was the Author of the little Treatise I am mentioning, was of an infirm Constitution, till about Forty, when by obstinately persisting in an exact Course of Temperance, he recover'd a perfect State of Health; insomuch that at fourscore he published his Book, which has been translated into *English* under the Title of *Sure and certain Methods of attaining a long and healthy Life*. He lived to give a Third o[r] Fourth Edition of it; and after having passed his Hundredth Year, died without Pain or Agony, and like one who falls asleep. The Treatise I mention, has been taken notice of by several eminent Authors, and is written with such a Spirit of Chearfulness, Religion, and good Sense, as are the natural Concomitants of Temperance and Sobriety. The Mixture of the old Man in it, is rather a Recommendation than a Discredit to it." For centuries, this passage accompanies translations of Cornaro.

22 Axon dates the first at 1704, the fourth he says "without editor's name, was published by the same bookseller in 1727" (p. 124). The fifth he says is a new version, but he misunderstood.

Precepts for the Preservation of Health, Life and Happiness, Medical and Moral by the illustrious doctor Clement Carlyon,[23] who, while understanding the inevitable changes to the times, judged Cornaro's rules still useful, at least for the well-to-do:

> Is it [[the Italian way]] applicable to England at the present time? It was so at the beginning of the last Century, according to the editor of the edition of Cornaro's Life of which I have availed myself. But now, in the middle of the nineteenth, is it so? Not to the same extent; but, even now, how great is the number of persons who die yearly from the effects of intemperance! I here allude more particularly to persons well to do in the world. (35)

In 1740 the version by Jones reappears – with his name as translator – as a third edition in Dublin;[24] in 1753 an edition comes out in Edinburgh,[25] revived with a slightly modified title by a different publisher in Edinburgh in 1768, and continued on to its 25th reprinting in 1777.[26] With respect to the *princeps*, the only novelty consists in having shortened the *Preface*, at the same time it gives the complete article by Addison. The edition of 1768 will be reproduced as is, but without being acknowledged by [A.B.] Air in 1811.[27]

The fame of Cornaro does not end in Europe: in 1787 his book crosses the ocean and finds a ready and enthusiastic welcome among American physicians, including some of the most famous exponents of the Harvard Medical School, such as Benjamin Waterhouse and Charles

---

23 By Clement Carlyon, M.D., late Fellow of Pembroke College, Cambridge (London, 1859). Cornaro's text covers pp. 163–235. Carlyon considers Cornaro's work the most indicative of expressing "the pith and virtual spirit" of all the treatises written up to then on the topic, and its author "a bright example of the good effect of a temperate diet, on which he lays the greatest stress, without losing sight of such important auxiliaries as healthy air and exercise, and a well regulated mind" (p. 32).

24 *Sure and Certain [M]ethods of attaining* (…). Made English by W.J. Jones (…). The third Edition. To which is prefix'd, Mr. Addison's account and recommendation of this book, etc. (Dublin, Printed by Richard Gunne, 1740).

25 (Printed by Ruddiman jun. and Company and sold by all Bookseller in Town. M.DCC. LIII). Cf. Axon, p. 124.

26 *Sure Methods of attaining a Long and Healthful Life.* By Lewis Cornaro. Translated from the Italian by W. Jones, A.B. The Twenty fifth Edition (Edinburgh: Printed by A. Donaldson, and sold at his shops in London and Edinburgh. MDCCLXXVII).

27 *Sure Methods of attaining a Long and Healthful Life.* Written originally in Italian, By Lewis Cornaro, A Noble Venetian, when near an hundred years old. Translated into English, by W. Jones, A.B. (Air: Printed by Wilson & Paul, 1811).

Chauncy. As soon as news spreads that the publisher George J. Osborne of Portsmouth intends to publish the treatise, Benjamin Waterhouse, "the astute young professor of medicine in the newly developed Harvard Medical School," writes to the publisher extolling the booklet – which he had brought with him from England – and recounting the effect that it had on his venerated professor Chauncy:

> I lent *Cornaro* to my venerable friend. The late *Doctor Chauncy*, who was sur-prized to find had never seen the work. When he returned it, he told me, he had read it again and again with more pleasure than any book of the kind he ever met with; for, says he, in my younger days I injured my con-stitution by severe study as much as *Cornaro* did by debaucheries, and as every wise man should be his own physician, I endeavoured to find out the causes of these depredations in my frame, and apply the remedy; and when I was assured that my eating, exercise and my habit of close thinking were disproportionate, I began to reform, and actually adopted the very method pursued by the noble Venetian, merely by consulting my own feelings, and without knowing any one had done so before me. In short, my plan of living was like *Cornaro's*, and my success the same; I now, says he, live as regular as the sun in the firmament, and if I eat a drachm weight more of flesh than usual, I feel it injure my system and cloud my faculties.[28]

The translation in the American printing is still that of Jones, but the sixth London edition, from which it was supposedly taken, turns out to be – at least for the moment – nonexistent. Perhaps it was a trick to avoid paying publishing rights or to ennoble in a certain sense the edition itself; the fact remains that the title has no corroboration in the long suc-cession of English prints.

Apart from the Air reprint in 1811, the Jones version will not be is-sued in its entirety during the nineteenth century, and will serve only to

---

28 *Benjamin Waterhouse on Luigi Cornaro's "Long and Healthful Life" with the test [sic] of The First American Edition. Portsmouth, New Hampshire,* 1788. Henry R. Viets, M.D. *Curator,* Boston Medical Library (Boston, Privately Printed, MCMLVI).

   The title for Cornaro: *The Probable Way of attaining a Lon[g] and Healthful Life; with the means of correcting a bad Constitution, &c.* Written originally in Italian by Lewis Cornaro, A Noble Venetian, When he was near an Hundred Years of Age. The Sixth Edition. (London, printed: Portsmouth, re-printed by George Jerry Osborne, and to be sold at his Office, near the State-House, M.DCC.LXXXVIII). In an appendix: "The case of Mr. Thomas Wood, a miller, of Billericary, in the county of Essex, England," extracted from *Medical Transactions,* vol. II.

integrate the one by White for the texts found in the appendix. It will return instead in this [20th] century with two complete editions, one in 1907 for the publisher J. Thomas of London, the other, a declared revival of the preceding one, at Nottingham in 1923.[29] Another edition, with a text much reworked and often summarized, appears in London in 1921 together with two brief works by Thomas Walker.[30] In none of the three is the translator cited.

We have seen how Jones boasts of his own distinction in respect to the translation by George Herbert, who in any case he does not name, and its fidelity in regard to the original. It is understandable enough: there is no doubt that his version is linguistically more modern and consists of all four discourses by Cornaro, except that it is not at all based on the original Italian but on the French translation by Mr. D. de Premont that appeared in Paris in 1701,[31] from which it also derives the supporting texts at the end, that is, the letter by the Nun (*Lettre d'une Religieuse de Padoue, Petite-Nièce de*

---

29 *Sure and Certain Methods of attaining a Long and Healthful Life* (…). Published by J. Thomas, 355, City Road, London, n.d., but in 1907 according to catalogues from the British Museum and the Bodleian. There is a preface by T.R. Allinson.

In 1923 C. J. Welton decided to reintroduce this edition: "In reference to the work by Cornaro, many editions of this famous work have been published during the past 100 years. The last edition was issued some 20 years ago by a very dear old friend of mine, Mr. J. Thomas, of City Road, London. I purchased the entire edition, which is now entirely sold out (…). It is a good book, and should be in the hands of every thoughtful person. It will well repay them for the reading" (pages not numbered). The publication presents two different titles: on the cover, *Cornaro's great work on Long Life Sure Methods. By one who lived over one hundred years.* Preface by C.J. Welton Author of "Marriage and Its Mysteries." (Published by C.J. Welton, Medical Hall, Nottingham; on the inside: New Edition, 1923). *Sure and Certain Methods of Attaining a Long and Healthful Life with means of correcting a bad constitution etc.* Written originally in Italian by Lewis Cornaro, A Noble Venetian, when he was near a Hundred Years of Age. And made English. (Published by C.J. Welton, Medical Hall, Nottingham).

30 *The Art of attaining high Health* by Thomas Walker, M.A. a learned Barrister at law. Together with *Aristology, or the Art of Dining* By the same Author. As also *A sure Method of attaining a Long Life* written originally in the Italian tongue by Signior Lewis Cornaro, a noble Venetian, and now in English. (London, Philip Allan & Co., MCMXXI). The Cornaro text is on pages 183–271.

31 This had also been noted by Axon, who, confounding the second edition of 1704 with that of the first, traced it back to a French version of 1703. Only the reprint in Amsterdam has this date. Not having been able to view the French *princeps*, we have based our comparison on the later publication: *De la Sobriété e de ses avantages, ou Le vrai moyen de se conserver dans une santé parfaite jusqu'à l'âge le plus avancé.* Traduction Nouvelle des Traités de *Lessius* & de *Cornaro* sur la vie sobre. (A Salerne, Et se trouve a Paris Chez Cailleau, Imprimeur-Libraire, rue Saint-Severin, M.DCC.LXXXII). The

Louis Cornaro), the passage of de Thou (*Extrait du trente-huitième Livre des Histoires de M. le Président de Thou, sur l'an* 1566),[32] that of Cardano already cited and, finally, *Moyens sûrs and faciles de remédier à divers accidens de la vie*; the texts that were reproduced in almost all later editions, with a clear preference for the Nun's letter, which still appears in 1935.

With respect to the French text, the Jones one is faithfully literal: the discourse straightforward and even, the "realism" of the admonitions and language that captivate the English reader so much are already all in the French version, which, though substantially faithful, is quite liberal and tends to stray somewhat. Let us look at an example:

> Certa cosa è che l'uso ne gli huomeni con il tempo si converte in natura sforzandogli a usar quello che s'usa, sia bene o male. Parimente vediamo in molte cose haver l'usanza più forza, che la ragione, che questo non si può negare: anzi bene speso si vede che usando un buono, et praticando con un cattivo di buono che era si fa cativo, si vede ancora il contrario cioè, che sì come facilmente la buona usanza in ria si converte, così ancora la ria ritorna

---

title in the foreword is *L'Art de vivre dans une Santé parfaite, jusqu'à l'âge le plus avancé.* The title for Cornaro: *De la vie sobre e réglée, ou L'art de vivre longtems dans une parfaite santé.* Traduit de l'italien de Louis Cornaro, Noble Vénitien. Nouvelle Édition. Augmentée de la manière de corriger un mauvais tempérament; de jouir d'une félicité parfaite jusqu'à l'âge le plus avancé, & de ne mourir que par la consommation de l'humide radical usé par une extrême veillesse.

That we are still dealing with the version by Mr. D. de Premont appears in the "Préface" by the new publisher: "Il y a près de quatre-vingt ans, qu'ils furent traduits en notre Langue; & l'on peut dire à la louange du Traducteur, que pour un tems aussi reculé, on ne pouvoit guères mieux écrire. A la réserve de quelques termes qui ne sont plus d'usage, cette Traduction, toute ancienne qu'elle est, pourroit encore passer. L'Auteur de cell-ci n'a seu qu'après l'avoir achevée, qu'il y en eût une ancienne; mais la sincérité ne lui permet point de ne pas avouer, que quand même il l'auroit sçu, avant de l'entreprendre, cela n'eût pas empêché qu'il ne l'eût entreprise. Cette ancienne Traduction ne se trouvoit presque plus. Cet Ouvrage méritoit d'ailleurs une nouvelle forme, qui en réveillât le goût. Et plusieurs personnes souhaitoient cette forme nouvelle" (pp. VIII–IX); furthermore, repeated is the *Approbation de Monsieur Burlet, de l'Académie Royale des Sciences, & Médecin de la Faculté de Paris, du 18 Mars 1698,* which appears at the end of the volume. Cf. J.Ch. Brunet, *Manuel de Libraire et de l'Amateur de Livres* (Copenhague, 1966), T. II, [p.] 275. A curiosity: on page 164, in the margin, we find a note written by a former reader who calculated Cornaro's ounces in grams: 12 oz. = 375 g, 14 oz. = 440 g, 16 oz. = 500 g.

32 It is the *Historia suis temporis* by Jacques Auguste de Thou (1553–1617), written in CXXXVIII [138] books, of which the first [eighteen] appeared in Paris in 1604 and the complete edition in 1620. It is impossible to pinpoint here the edition from which the passage was taken. Cf. Brunet, [*Manuel de Libraire ...*,] T. V, [pp.] 842–3.

in buona: perché poi vediamo che questo malvagio, che prima era buono praticherà con un buono e lo ritornerà buono, e ciò non prociede se non per la forza del'uso la qual è veramente grande (I° discorso, inizio, 171a);

Rien n'est plus certain, que l'habitude passe aisément on nature, & qu'elle a sur tous le corps un extrême pouvoir; elle a même souvent sur l'esprit plus d'autorité que la raison. Le plus honnête homme, en fréquentant des libertins, oublie peu-à-peu les maximes de probité qu'il a succées avec le lait, & s'abandonne à des vices qu'il voit continuellement pratiquer. Est-il assez heurex pour être séparé de cette mauvaise société, & pour se trouver souvent en meilleure compagnie, la vertu triomphe à son tour; il reprend insensiblement sa sagesse qu'il avoit abandonnée. Enfin tous les changemens que nous voyons arriver dans le tempérament, dans la conduite & dans les moeurs de la plûpart des hommes, n'ont presque point d'autres principes que la force de l'habitude. (141–2)

Nothing is more certain than that Custom becomes a second Nature, and has a great Influence upon our Bodies. Nay, it has too often more Power over the Mind, than Reason it self. The honestest Man alive, in keeping company with Libertines, by degrees forgets the Maxims of Probity which be had imbibed from the very Breast, and gives himself the Loose in those Vices which he sees practis'd. If he be so happy as to relinquish that bad Company, and to meet with Better, Virtue will triumph in its Turn; and he insensibly resumes the Wisdom which he had abandoned. In a word, all the Alterations which we perceive in the Temper, Carriage, and Manner of most men, have scarce any other Foundation but the force and prevalency of Custom. (1–2)

Furthermore, Jones – but he had already warned us in his preface – modifies the text by censoring everything said against Lutheran doctrine; for example, the "*tre mali costumi*" [three bad habits] that Cornaro said were introduced into Italy (i.e., flattery and ceremonies, Lutheranism, crapula) remain in the French:

Je compte pour le premier l'adulation & les cérémonies. La second est l'hérésie de Luther, qui commence à faire du progrès. La troisième est l'yvrognerie & la gourmandise. (142)

But for the English – and so it will remain in all [their] translations except for the first one by White and the American edition of 1903 – there are only two:

(…) the first I reckon to be Flattery and Cerimonies [*sic*]; and the second, Intemperance both in Eating and Drinking. (2)

In the sequence of English and American publishers of Cornaro, Benjamin White is the only one to consider offering to readers a rigorous and complete translation to the extent of including the original Italian with his text:

> This useful work was translated some years ago into English, under the title of *Sure and certain methods of attaining a long and healthy life.* The translator seems rather to have made use of a French version than of the Italian original; he has likewise omitted several passages of the Italian, and the whole is rather a paraphrase than a translation. This has induced us to give the public an exact and faithful version of that excellence performance, from the Venice edition in 8vo, in the year 1620. (*Preface,* vi–vii)[33]

And it is also the only one to limit religious scruples to this brief note on the incriminated passage against Lutheranism:

> The author writes with the prejudice of a zealous Roman Catholic against the doctrine of the Reformation, which he here distinguishes by the name of Lutheranism. This was owing to the artifices of the Romish clergy in those days, by whom the reformed religion was misrepresented, as introductive of licentiousness and debauchery. (2)

The introductory information on the life of Cornaro is drawn by White from the Nun's letter, which, however, he does not cite. Moreover, he brings back the passage by Addison and erroneously adds in a note that the first complete edition of the *Vita sobria* is the one from Padua dated 1558. Nothing, instead, is said about the author of the new version whom we can assume to be that same White.

This edition is revived, identical in title and text but missing the original Italian, at Glasgow in 1770;[34] it then reappears corrected – meaning

---

33 *Discourses on a Sober and Temperate Life.* By Lawis Cornaro, a Noble Venetian. Translated from the Italian original. (London: Printed for Benjamin White, at Horace's Head, In Fleet-Street. MDCCLXVIII).
   Discorsi della Vita Sobria, Del Sig. Luigi Cornaro. Ne' quali con l'esempio de se stesso dimostra con quai mezzi possa l'huomo conservarsi sano insin'all'ultima vecchiezza. Nuovamente ristampati, & dedicati All'Illustriss. e Revendiss. Sig. Mons. Marco Cornaro Vescovo di Padoua. Con Licentia de' Superiori. (In Venetia, Appresso Marc'Antonio Brogiollo. MDCXX. In Londra, Ristampato da Benjamino White. MDCCLXVIII).
34 Glasgow: Printed for Robert Urie. MDCCLXX.

censored – in London in 1798,[35] and will be included in the treatise by Sir John Sinclair, *The Code of Health and Longevity* of 1807.[36]

Sinclair, an admirer of Cornaro, whom he considers "another memorable example of the efficacy of rules," nevertheless shows he is little convinced in regard to his diet, so much so as to rouse the ire of another famous physician, Carlyon, who rebuts as follows:

> I have always thought that Lewis Cornaro's Autobiography comprises, in spirit, all that can be said respecting 'The Methods of attaining a Long and Healthful Life,' as well as of the value of its attainment.
>
> Sir John Sinclair, in his "Code of Health and Longevithy," has gone into details which are so infinite in variety, as to become perplexing; and he has done Cornaro injustice in saying, that, "on the whole, too much stress has been laid on the doctrines of Cornaro," apparently misled by some remarks of Feyjoo, that "God did not create Lewis Cornaro to be a rule for all mankind in what they were to eat or drink." I know little more of Feyjoo than that he was a Spanish Benedictine Friar. The beauty and excellence of Cornaro's Code consists in the good sense and liberality of its entire tenour: he tells us what good he derived from a particular diet, but he guards especially against the imputation of wishing to restrict others to the same measure with himself. I have, therefore, thought it well to let Cornaro again speak for himself, believing that a Treatise can scarcely come too often before the public of which Addison long ago said, that "It is written with such a spirit of cheerfulness, Religion and good Sense, as are the natural Concomitants of Temperance and Sobriety; the Mixture of the old Man in it, is rather a Recommendation than a Discredit."[37]

---

35 *Discourses on a Sober and Temperate Life. By Lewis Cornaro, a Noble Venetian. Wherein is demonstrated, by his own Example, the Method of Preserving Health to extreme Age.* Translated from the Italian Original. A new Edition, corrected, to which is added, *Physic of the Golden Age, a Fragment.* (London: Cadell & Davies, 1798). Also censored are the passages on Lutheranism.

36 R.H. Sir John Sinclair, *The Code of Health and Longevity; or, A general view of the Rules and Principles calculated for the preservation of Health, and the attainement of a long Life.* (London 1807), vol. III. Sinclair refers to an edition of 1799 that is unfamiliar to us (cf. Axon, p. 127). In successive editions of the *Code*, the text by Cornaro does not appear but the notes remain.

37 C. Carlyon, *Precepts for the Preservation of Health ...*, pp. 165–6. Sinclair had said: "On the whole, too much stress seems to be laid on the doctrines of Cornaro. Feyjoo remarks, that God did no[t] create Lewis Cornaro to be a rule for all mankind in what they were to eat and drink. The learned Jesuit Lessius, who translated the Treatise of

We again find the version by White in Boston, in 1814.[38] Two years later it reappears in London but only with the first, second, and fourth discourses.[39] Some years later, an almost inexhaustible succession of editions and reprints emerge, from among which they are not always easily untangled: in 1820 we have given as the 32nd edition a kind of "sandwich" in which is found: the *Preface* by White of 1768, the article by Addison, the four discourses reworked and modernized by White with the titles taken in a somewhat modified form from Jones, the Nun's letter, and the sayings and maxims. All preceded by a portrait of Cornaro – reversed with respect to the original in the Pitti Gallery* – where we read "Lewis Cornaro at the age of 100 years."[40] From this edition are derived the one published in the review *The Pamphleteer* (1821,1822),[41] indicated as the 33rd printing, the 34th of 1822, the 36th of 1826, all by Anderson of London. But [editions] also derived are the impossible 40th of 1821, the 45th of 1823, the 53rd of 1825, the 54th perhaps of

---

Cornaro from Italian into Latin, was so strongly persuaded by it, that he had bound himself under the same restrictions. He, however, lived only to the age of seventy-nine, and that with many disorders which he laboured under. To one man, like Cornaro, who lived an hundred years with such strict diet, we may oppose a great number of others, who have lived much longer, without all these scruples. His constitution required such abstinence, which few others might be able to bear. *Father Feyjoo's Rules of Preserving Health*, [p.] 82. Cornaro tells us, that in order to preserve his health, he not only resolved to restrict himself, as to the quantity of his liquid and solid food, but carefully to avoid cold, fatigue, grief, watchings, and every other excess, that could hurt his health. How could the business of the world be carried on, if every man, like Cornaro, were to begin following that system at the fortieth year of his age?" [*Father Feyjoo's* …,] 3rd edition, (London: B. McMillan, Bow-Street, Covent-Garden, 1816), p. 195 note. Feyjoo is Benito Jerónimo Feyjoo y Montenero (1676–1764), General Abbot of the Benedictines, author of *Theatro crítico universal* (Madrid 1726–1739), 8 vols.

38 *Discourses etc.* (Boston: Thomas B. Wait & Sons, 1814). The British Museum catalogue refers to a prior edition of 1806 which was not found, unless it is the one by Sinclair.

39 *A Guide t[o] Health and Long Life* (…) (London: J. Brettel, for Clark, 1816).

 * [Cornaro's portrait (c.1560 to 1565) in the Galleria Palatina at the Pitti Palace (Florence, Italy), is by Tintoretto (Jacopo Comin, 1519–1594).]

40 *Sur[e] Methods of attaining a Long and Healthful Life: with the Means of correcting a bad Constitution.* By Lewis Cornaro. Translated from Italian. Thirty-second Edition. (London: Printed for John Anderson, 40, West Smithfield; and J. Smith, 163, Strand. 1820).

41 Vol. XIII, (1821), pp. 495–522; XIX (1822), pp. 135–60. No mention is made of the edition from which the text was taken.

1830, all by G. A. Williams of Cheltenham;[42] and again, the 55th of 1832 for F.E. Bingley of Leeds. In 1872, under a slightly different title, a 30th edition is issued in London, which, with respect to its predecessors, is missing the portrait but the maxims are reinstated.[43]

Whether the edition numbers are true or not, the fact still remains that never have so many appeared as in that century. The discussions and debates among physicians in regard to Cornaro's rules certainly favoured the growing fame of this Paduan centenarian among the public at large, and many, persuaded by his example, followed his rules. But it was always a matter of individual choice until the arrival of C.F. Carpenter, who – sensing a business opportunity – thought well about taking advantage of the occasion. So it was in 1879 that Mr. Carpenter, proprietor of the hotel "The South Devon Health Resort," published it at his own expense, but only with the points relevant to the diet found in the version by White. He was also careful to remove the passage by Cardano, so as not to raise any doubts, and replaced White's "preface" with his own, in which, among other things, we read:

> The chief object of the proprietor is to restore the health of his patients as quickly as possible, so that, while everything necessary for comfort is supplied, enervating luxuries are, as far as possible, avoided. And, as he knows from experience the great importance of a *well-regulated dietary* in the restoration of health, he has devoted considerable attention to that subject, and the particular condition of each patient will, in this respect, be carefully studied. Nothing is provided but what is one of the *purest quality*, and it may be mentioned that all the wheat, from which the bread, etc., is made, is cleaned and ground in a special manner for the establishment. (3–4)[44]

---

42 The title is identical to the one of 1820, [Cornaro's] portrait therein is a rough copy. After the number of the edition, we have: Cheltenham: Printed for G.A. Williams, Librarian, and Longman and Co.; and G. & W.E. Whittaker, London. The year follows. James Bennet, Printer, Tewkesbury. In these editions, the *Maxims* are substituted with *Aphorisms and Maxims of celebrated Physicians, &c. in corroboration of the Opinions of Cornaro.*

43 *Sure Methods of attaining a Long and Healthful Life, with the means of Correcting a bad Constitution.* Translated from the Italian of Lewis Cornaro, a noble Venetian, when he was nearly a hundred years of age. Thirtieth Edition. (Henry Renshaw, 356, Strand, London. 1872). The British Museum catalogue refers to the 1832 edition, the Bodleian to that of 1821.

Business was not to go badly for Mr. Carpenter, who republished the text in 1882 and again in [18]94. At the back of this last edition we find two pages of entertaining publicity. On the first, the qualities of Carpenter's resort are celebrated:

The South Devon Health Resort. Turkish and other Baths. Electricity, Massage. Is strongly recommended to all needing rest and pleasant and healthful change. It is one of the loveliest spots in the county, and "has all the comfort and charm of a gentleman's country home." Beautiful private grounds, lawn tennis. The residence stands 200 feet above sea-level, yet is well sheltered from the north-east by Haldon Down, 800 feet. It has a full south aspect, with splendid view across the Teign Valley and estuary. To the west lies Dartmoor. The climate is probably unsurpassed in England for winter and spring. Teignmouth is the nearest station, 2½ miles. For terms and testimonials apply to C.F. Carpenter, Bishop's Teignton, near Teignmouth.

On the second, there is a cough syrup:

How to Stop a Cough! / By hundreds who have done it and can prove the / fact if you wish. Simply take / Wellington's / Celebrated Bekosine / The Great Cough & Cold Cure / in conjunction with his / noted family aperient pills / and you will add one more to the number. / In Bottles a 1–1½ and 2/9 each, of all Chemists; or Post Free for 1/4 and 3. From F. Wellington, The Chemist, Parade, Taunton (formerly Hitchcock). Wholesale London Agents: Barclay and Edwards.

The White version reappears with the usual portrait in an American printing of 1912, which is passed off as an English translation of 1809, which in turn is based on a Venetian edition of 1612. It brings back the *preface* of 1768, the passage from the "Spectator," and the four

---

44 Cover title: *How to regain Health and live 100 years. By one who did it.* Inside title: *How to live a hundred Years by One who has done it,* Translated from the Italian of Lewis Cornaro. (London, Simpkin Marshall & Company, 1879). At the end of the "Contents" is a "Prospectus of the South Devon Health Resort Bishop's-Teignton Situated between Dawlish and Torquay About two miles from the sea. C.F. Carpenter, Proprietor." The second edition is from 1882 (Axon, p. 125).

discourses.[45] One year later there is another edition in London:[46] no mention is made of either the translator or the editor. After a brief introduction in which all the known Cornaro specialists are included, among whom were the Queen of Cyprus and a certain Lucrezia, whose literary successes are recounted – who is obviously Elena Lucrezia Cornaro Piscopia[*] – it then goes on to recount the life of Alvise, with information randomly taken from the Nun's letter and from de Thou without, in any case, citing them. The appendix is more interesting, being a reprint of the discussion held by the doctor Ernest Van Someren in 1901 before the Physiological Session of the British Medical Association.[47]

---

45 *Methods of attaining a long Life By Luigi Cornaro Wherein is Demonstrated by the Author's Own Example the Method of Preserving Health to Extreme Old Age.* Translated from the Italian of the Venice Edition of 1612. G.P. Putnam's Sons, New York and London, The Knickerbocker Press, n.d., but it is 1912 according to the date in the editor's note for the first American edition, in which among other things we read: "The treatise on *Health and Long Life* by the noble Venetian, Lewis Cornaro, has long been accepted as a Classic (...). We have utilised as the text for the present American Edition a translation prepared in London in 1809 (...). The interest is as keen in the twentieth century as it was in the sixteenth, in regard to any methods that may serve to strengthen health and to further the prospects of longevity. The methods followed by Cornaro and the recommendations and suggestions submitted by him can be compared to advantage with the teachings of authorities of the present day, such as Metchnikoff. The book is now presented to the American public, not only as a literary and scientific curiosity, but as a manual of practical instruction" (pp. III–IV).

46 *How Luigi Cornaro regained his healt[h] and lived 100 years. Together with An Introduction and an address by Dr. E. van Someren on Luigi Cornaro's Method.* Reprinted, by permission, from Mr. Horace Fletcher's book "The A. B.– Z of Our Own Nutrition." (London: Ewart, Seymour & Co., Ltd., Twelve Burleight St., Strand), n.d.

 * [Elena Lucrezia Cornaro Piscopia (1646–1684), born in Padua, religiously devout and exceptional for her encyclopedic knowledge, in 1637, at the age of thirty-two, became the first woman in the world documented for having been awarded a doctorate degree (*Magistra et Doctrix Philosophiae*). A consequent, however, was that women at the University of Padua, where she had earned that degree, were not allowed to take a doctorate exam for some 300 years to follow. Tributes to this remarkable person include a statue at her alma mater in Padua (twentieth century), a "massive" stained-glass window (1905) called the *Cornaro window* in the Thompson Memorial Library at Vassar College, and a mural of her on the wall of the Italian Room at the University of Pittsburgh overlooks the students. She is believed to have died of tuberculosis.]

47 Dr. van Someren asked: "Did Luigi Cornaro make use of a physiological process unknown to us, and of the value of which he himself was not cognizant? To live to an advanced age, must we be as temperate as he, reducing the quantity of our food to a minimum required by nature?" (pp. 69–9 [*sic*]). He then proceeds to speak on

Finally, we again find the White version in the most recent edition of Cornaro, in London in 1951. The editor, Harry Clements, does not say a word about the translation brought out by him and accepts, unquestioningly, the information on Cornaro's life provided by Anton Maria Graziani. With respect to the preceding editions, along with the letter to Barbaro, here he adds the one to Speroni on the death of Ruzzante.[48]

Quite a different case, within the history of those versions by Jones and White, is the edition that appeared at Philadelphia in 1796, which offers a successfully received condensation of the two. It is clear that no consideration was made of the original text, instead it has taken – at times faithfully, at times summarizing, and at other times eliminating – that which the Reverend Mason I. Weems held to be useful for his purpose: to provide through the teachings of Cornaro, [Benjamin] Franklin and Scott, an infallible guide to the reader.[49]

In contrast to the two versions examined above, the one that appeared in London toward the middle of the 1700s had scant success, but even it created some confusion. Axon cites a London printing of 1742 completely identical to that of 1743,[50] (in our view), minus the list of subscribers and the name of the translator, which in the first – still according

---

the importance of mastication, of a milk diet, and of "bacterial digestion," and he concludes that, if one can eat less and stay healthy, one should not, in any case, exaggerate: "The writer, bearing in mind the warning suggested by the Frenchman, whose donkey died as soon as he had reduced his food to a single wisp of straw, finds that he is taking less and less food. While his mind is open as to his arrival at the final diet of Luigi Cornaro, yet it is easily conceivable that living a similar life or retirement in a placid environment, it would be quite possible to do as he did. Hence the title of this paper and the queries at the commencement" (p. 85). The appendix is on pages 68–85.

48 *How to live one Hundred Years. The Famous Treatise written Four Hundred Years ago on Health and Longevity by Luigi Cornaro.* With an introduction by Harry Clements. (London: Health for all Publishing Company; First edition 1951). Cf., A.M. Graziani, *De vita Joannis Francisci Commendoni Cardinalis libri quatuor,* (Parisiis, apud S. Mabre Cramoisy, 1669), 1. I, Ch. IV.

49 *The Immortal Mentor: or, Man's unerring Guide to a Healthy, Wealthy, and Happy Life.* In three Parts. By Lewis Cornaro, Dr Franklin, and Dr Scott. (Philadelphia: Printed for the Rev. Mason L. Weems, by Francis and Robert Bailey, N. 116, High Street. 1976). Of Cornaro, only his discourses are given, which are followed by the appendix "Golden Rules of Health, selected from Hippocrates, Plutarch, and several other eminent Physicians and Philosophers." By B. Franklin, "The Way to Wealth, and Advice to a Young Tradesman"; by Scott, "A sure Guide to Happiness," and "On social Love."

50 *A Treatise of Health and Long Life, With the sure Means of attaining it, in Two Books.* The First by Leonard Lessius, The Second by Lewis Cornaro, A Noble Venetian. Translated

to Axon – turns out to be Timothy Smith, and in the second Thomas Smith. On this switch of names he chances upon a little mystery that is completely incongruous, since the 1743 printing also shows the name Timothy Smith, to which was added the qualification of Apothecary.[51] It is therefore a simple matter of a misreading. Axon again observed: "To make the matter still more complicated, the appearance of Timothy Smith in connection with the translation of Lessius had led to the occasional association of his name with the unknown 'T.S.' who wrote the introduction to the Cambridge 'Hygiasticon.' The version of Timothy Smith and Thomas Smith are identical, but that of the earlier 'T.S.' is quite distinct" (126–7). And here, the comparison is not understood, given that in the Cambridge edition, Cornaro was translated by George Herbert. In reality, the three figures bearing the same initials are the one person, that same T.S. – translator of Lessius in 1633 – who evidently also provided his own version of Cornaro but published the one by Herbert, which had been requested of him. That this is true is demonstrated by the same translation of the elusive Timothy Smith who slavishly follows the text by Lessius, copying the paragraph titles, the few additions and omissions. The patently obvious proof is actually in the passage already cited about the proverbs, for which the Latin translation of Lessius is given in a note. The only variation is the censoring in regard to Lutheranism. The name Timothy Smith is but a false play on the initials of the age-old translator: one of the many spirited inventions employed by the publishers, each and every time, for passing off as new things centuries old.

Some one hundred and fifty years must pass to find another original version following that of White, and it will be the American one published by William F. Butler of Milwaukee in 1903. This is a precise and complete edition of the four Discourses with a generous introduction, in which appears the inevitable passage by Addison and an appendix that includes, in addition to the history of the Cornaro family, the *Eulogy* by

---

into English, by Timothy Smith, Apothecary. (London: Printed for Charles Hitch, at the *Red Lyon*, in *Pater-nostrer Row*, James Leake in *Bath*, and William Flackton in *Canterbury*, 1743).

The title for Cornaro: *A Treatise of the Benefits of a Sober Life*. Written originally in Italian, by Lewis Cornaro, A Noble Venetian: Translated into Latin, by Leonard Lessius, And now into English, by T.S. (London: Printed in the Year M.DCC.XLIII).

51 Axon (pp. 125–6). He also speaks of a copy dated 1767 at the British Museum, but it is nowhere to be found in the catalogue.

Bartolomeo Gamba and the essay on Cornaro's villas by Emilio Lovarini. However, it lacks any information on the original text from which the version was taken, although presumably it is traceable to the Venetian version of 1816 by Gamba. In regard to the translation, only [the following] is given to us in the *Preface*: "A carefully revised version of his celebrated treatise, made by able translators, is here presented." A work of many hands, therefore, which takes nothing away from the fidelity of the text or its linguistic fluency.[52]

After this lengthy evaluation of editions, reprints, judgments and discussions that have kept the name of Cornaro alive almost four hundred years, we might conclude that the diet is worthy of a similar glory. But there remains the doubt that, if the good Cornaro had not lied about his own age, he too would have ended up among the crowd of advice-giving essayists destined to go unheeded for having had the misfortune of not dying centenarians, or presumed as such. The fat miller of Essex is not gullible: he enthusiastically accepts to follow an example of proven success; and the clever resort owner of Devon capitalizes one hundred fifty years later on the same point. "Most readers," – comments Axon – "even if they hesitate to adopt Cornaro's rules, find pleasure in listening to the good old man who takes such frank delight in his healthy age, and has such sure conviction that this method is open to everyone, and will prove a remedy in the most desperate cases. We see him in his pleasant gardens surrounded by his grandchildren, enjoying their musical exercises, and

---

52 *The Art of Living Long*. A new and improved English Version of the Treatise of the Celebrated Venetian Centenarian Louis Cornaro. With essay by Joseph Addison, Lord Bacon, and Sir William Temple. (Milwaukee: William F. Butler, 1903).

The existing copy in the Radcliffe Science Library at Oxford contains a signed letter by Butler indicating his donation of the book to the Bodleian, the entry of presentation for the work and a curious booklet without author, place or date, intitled: *An abridged list of Works containing articles on Louis Cornaro and his writing*. Unfortunately the promise remains in the title in that it is only a list of encyclopedias, dictionaries, etc., in which Cornaro is named, the libraries where his works can be found, and a shorter list of notes on "Medical Works" that in the final analysis are medical dictionaries.

According to Axon, an American edition exists that precedes it: "In the Surgeon-General's Library at Washington there is a copy of 'The Discourses and Letters of Louis Cornaro on a sober and temperate life; with a biography of the author by Piero Maroncelli, with notes and an appendix by John Burdett. (Twenty-fifth thousand). (New York: Fowler and Wells. [1842])' This I have not seen," (pp. 127–8).

The Lovarini essay is "Le ville edificate da Alvise Cornaro," in *L'Arte* ..., II pp. 191–212.

he himself singing because he has 'a clearer and louder pipe than at any other period of life.' This, with the composition of a comedy (…) and more serious essays, scientific and literary, intended for the benefit of the commonwealth, were the recreations of his old age. As a teacher of 'plain living and high thinking,' Cornaro has still a useful mission" (129).

Perhaps now that even Cornaro has been shown in more human terms there will be no more talk of a "useful mission," but of an old man's obsession. What a shame, another legend gone.

[Marisa Milani 1980]

Selected Terminology

The following notes on selected terminology – by no means definitive – serve both to inform Cornaro's writings and to encourage further investigation by the reader.

Alvise: Aluvise = Alvise. Cornaro's name is a variation on the Latin *Clovis*. Other renderings would include: Ludwig, Ludvig, Lodovico, Ludovico, Luigi, Aloysius, Lewis, Louis, or Luis, and so on.

Animo: from the Latin *animus,* it is the "soul of Man as the foundation of the intellectual and moral faculties, of sentiment [the senses], of the will (and indicates, with respect to 'anima,' a more particular and limited aspect of the human spirit)" *Dictionary of the Italian Language* (UTET), *s.v.* p. 485. The sense of *animo* can vary, and signifies the "human" soul of reason, emotion, perception, character, the will, or intention, moral virtue (among other faculties and processes). Certain phrases in Italian are now colloquial: *nel profondo dell animo* [deep in one's heart, or soul]; *perdersi d' animo* [to lose heart, to be discouraged]; *forza d'animo* [willpower, fortitude, intent]; *stato d'animo* [emotional state, feelings, state of mind, etc]. On further consideration of this much debated and challenging term, see the essay by K.V. Wilkes, "*Psuchē* versus Mind," in *Essays on Aristotle's De Anima* (pp. 109–27), in which it is argued that the modern use of consciousness and mind to signify psuchē (psyche > *anima* (soul) > *animo*) has been "[a]dopted and reinforced by the British Empiricists, this picture is one with which philosophers in the English-language tradition have been struggling ever since. By and large it did not impress writers and poets … and was not supreme in philosophy in continental Europe. But it drastically coloured the birth of scientific psychology" (K.V. Wilkes, ibid., p. 115). Also see Noga

Arikha's estimation that – despite a modern signifier of "mind" – "The science of psychology as we know it today was born in the nineteenth century, but when the term [*animo*] is used within an earlier context, it should be taken to mean the study of the soul," in "A Note on Terminology" in *Passions and Tempers,* page not numbered). Also see below: *Anima, Psuchē, Soul,* or *Spirit.*

Bread: Cornaro writes on the merits of plain bread in his "ode" to it (*Sober* ..., pp. 113-14, 161). "The social significance of bread in the Renaissance," writes Ken Albala, "is no less complicated than our own. According to standard theory, the best bread is made of hard wheat, well milled and bolted, made into a dough properly salted, kneaded, well risen, well baked in an oven, and thoroughly cooled. Thus anything of mixed flour, containing too much bran, unsalted, flat, burnt, or hot is inferior." He goes on to say that there was a "general preference for whiter bread with little bran. Being more expensive, it was naturally a sign of status. [Michele] Savonarola, as we might expect assigns bread made of the *fiore di formento* [flour of wheat or pollen], made without any bran, to princes and great masters. Its opposite, made with a great deal of bran, is 'bread for dogs.' ... Savonarola's estimation of bread is indeed polar. White bread versus bran bread reflects an essentially two-tiered system" (K. Abala, *Eating Right* ..., pp. 196–7). To extend the flour or bran, the economically poorer consumer added ingredients such as barley, rye, chestnuts, or beans. "Whole wheat bread was probably more nutritious than white bread, or at least the roughage promoted good digestion, but stone-ground flours also contained minute particles of stone which seriously wore down people's teeth" (K. Albala, *Food in Early Modern Europe* ..., p. 22). On the social variances of bread, also see, Robert Jütte, *Poverty and Deviance* ...; and Piero Camporesi's provocative study of the social role of bread, and some of its additives, which caused the consumer harm or to become "crazed," or "dazed" (*darnel*), in his *Il Pane selvaggio* (translated as *Bread of Dreams* ..., by David Gentilcore, 1989).

Cause: As noted by Marsilio Ficino, the four causes of creation, according to Thierry Chartres, consist of "the efficient cause (the power of God), the formal cause (the wisdom of God) and the final cause (the goodness of God); the material cause being the four elements," M. Ficino, *Letters of Marsilio Ficino* (Vol. 2, p. 92, note 21:4).

Coitus: For Cornaro, (following Plato, Galen, and others), the sensual (sensuality) or that which is based on the appetites of the senses – is not a desirable trait in a man, since it fosters unrestrained and unchaste behaviour (*incontinenza*) that compromises his ability to reason. "Galen" – much admired by Cornaro – "was cautious about sexual relations. He advised his readers not to be like dumb animals but to judge by experience what proved injurious to them. He felt that although some men were greatly injured by having sexual intercourse, and others remained uninjured until old men, most men should have sex in moderation. In another work he advocated that men not only practice self control over their anger but also clear themselves of voluptuous eating, carnal lust, drunkenness, excessive curiosity, and envy, in order to achieve the peak of temperance. This concept of moderation appears throughout the Middle Ages along with an emphasis on celibacy, as is evident in that most popular of Salernitan medical compilations, the eleventh-century *Regimen sanitatis*" (Vern L. Bullough, "Medieval Medical and Scientific Views of Women," in *Viator - Center for Medieval and Renaissance Studies,* ed. Lynne White Jr. [Los Angeles: University of California Press, 1973], Vol. 4, pp. 485–501, at p. 498). The "radical moisture" for Avicenna (Ibn Sinā, 980–1037) – Islamic philosopher and physician – was of man's semen (seminal, the fourth moisture). N. Arikha explains: "Excessive sexual intercourse could undermine the intellect: it 'drains the spirits, especially the more subtle ones, it weakens the brain, and it ruins the stomach and the heart.' Hippocrates was right to claim it was like epilepsy; and Avicenna was right to say, 'If any sperm should flow away through sexual intercourse beyond that which nature tolerates, it is more harmful than if forty times as much blood should pour forth'" (*Passions* ..., p. 124). Also see *Sober* ..., p. 82n24, and see below: *Semen.*

Complexion: Nancy Siraisi states: "The humors filled two important functions in the body's economy. In the first place, they were essential to nutrition. Indeed, in Galenic physiology, the blood, incorporating within it the other humors, *is* the body's nutrition.... Avicenna's account is brief and clear: ingested food, having been transformed into chyle in the stomach, is subsequently transported to the liver and there concocted (literally, 'cooked') into blood, the two biles, and phlegm. Various stages of concoction purify the blood of superfluities which are excreted, and ultimately, part of the blood is refined into semen. Most of the blood, however, is used up in nourishing every part of the body. Hence, the parts of the body were said to be generated from the humours. ¶ Second, the humours were in a special way the vehicle of complexion.... But in addition, the four humours were collectively the means whereby an individual's overall complexional balance was maintained or altered. Hence the balance of humours was held to be responsible for psychological as well as physical disposition" (N. Siraisi, *Medieval and Early Renaissance Medicine* ..., p. 106). Also see N. Arikha, *Passions* ..., (2007); and see below: *Humours,* and *Temperament.*

Continence: One of the four Cardinal Virtues (along with Prudence, Justice, and Fortitude). In terms of virtue, it is "a holding back, repression (of torments, desires, etc.) ... Self-restraint in the matter of sexual appetite, displayed either by due moderation or ... by entire abstinence" *OED, s.v.* It can also signify chastity. Also see above: *Coitus.*

Elements: Empedocles (c. 492?–432? BCE), a philosopher born in Agrigentum, Sicily, held that the roots of things were Air, Water, Earth, and Fire, and that the two cosmic forces love (*philia*) and strife (*neikos*) could affect their interaction. To these four classical elements, Aristotle included "Ether" (aether), the celestial world of stars and planets as being the fifth element or essence, attributing the properties of hot or cold, dry or wet, to the four elements. Air is thus both hot and wet; water is cold and wet; earth is cold and dry; fire is hot and dry.

Humours: "A humour is literally a fluid – *humon* in Greek, (*h*)*umor* in Latin – and bodily humours are fluids within a living organism ... An excess of food or drink could cause a humoural imbalance, bringing about illness or, at worst, death" (N. Arikha, *Passions and Tempers* ..., p. xviii). The four humours are essential fluids manufactured in the body that regulate physiological functions. Although a complete theory of humours was not formulated at the time of the Hippocratic writers, they often referred to health as a balance of hot or cold and moist or dry properties, and some authors referred to specific humours. "The systematic description of four distinct fluids was first proposed by Galen, who described the humors in terms of elemental properties. Blood was described as a cold and moist humor, phlegm as cold and moist, choler (yellow bile) as hot and dry, and melancholy (black bile) as cold and dry" (K. Albala, *Eating Right* ..., pp. 48–9). The four humours are found in different proportions within the body, blood being the most abundant. The ratio of blood (air) is 4:1 greater than phlegm (water); 16:1 greater than choler (fire); and 64:1 greater than black bile (earth). "Perfect health, or 'eukrasia,' which is extremely rare, consists in maintaining this delicate proportional balance ... the balance of humours required much more than quantitative regulation. The internal physiological systems also had to be in optimal working order," (K. Albala, *Eating Right* ..., pp. 49–50). "Secondly, the humors were in a special way the vehicle of complexion.... But in addition, the four humors were collectively the means whereby an individual's overall complexional balance was maintained or altered. Hence the balance of humors was held to be responsible for psychological as well as physical disposition" (N. Siraisi, *Medieval and Early Renaissance Medicine* ..., p. 106). Also see above: *Complexion.*

Panatella: A very light and digestible soup of grated bread, suitable for the infirm. The word *panata* – at times, *panada* – in Italian, is the past tense of the verb *panare* (to coat food with grated bread), *panatella* being the diminuitive of *panata.* "La panata è una minestra fatta di pane raffermo sminuzzato o grattugiato e cotto in acqua, latte o brodo. Può essere condita a piacere" [Panata is a soup made of stale bread crumbled into pieces or grated and cooked in water, milk, or broth. It can be seasoned as desired] (M. Milani, *Orazione* ..., p. 66). Cf., Dizionario ..., UTET, Battaglia, *s.v.* Variations on this recipe can be found in Renaissance texts on health and eating. On recipes, ingredients, cooking implements, and techniques of sixteenth-century Italy, see *The "Opera" of Bartolomeo Scappi* (1570): *l'arte et prudenza d'un maestro cuoco.* Trans. with commentary Terence Scully (Toronto: University of Toronto Press, 2008); also on food items and utensils of the same Scappi, see for example, June di Schino and Furio Luccichenti, *Il cuoco segreto dei papi. Bartolomeo Scappi e la Confraternita dei cuochi e dei pasticierri* (Roma: Gangemi Editore, 2007).

Perturbation: an "agitation" located in the lower soul, or a disorder of the humours, derangement, or distemper (intemperance), which either tend towards good (joy) or to evil (hate, anger); for example, having to do with emotional perceptions in the sense of torments, but not out of desire. On Cicero's "Disputations," Robert E. Proctor writes: "The *Tusculan Disputations* consist of four dialogues concerning death, pain, mental anguish, and other 'perturbations' of the soul" (p. 64). "It is these turbulent motions which Cicero calls 'perturbations,' defining perturbation as 'an agitation of the soul (*animi commotio*) averse to reason, and against nature'" (R. Proctor, *Defining the Humanities* ..., p. 65). Also see below: *Spirit.*

Semen: Pythagoras (c. sixth century BCE) thought that semen drops from the brain, and to safeguard the intellect it is better to be continent (chaste) to retain the semen and nourish the brain. Alcmaeon of

Croton (c. sixth – fifth century BCE) speculated that semen is the product of brain substance, travelling from the brain, through the veins into the spinal cord, and from there to the testicles; see for example, J. Longrigg, *Greek Rational Medicine: Philosophy and Medicine from Alcmaeon to the Alexandrians* (1993). Semen was also thought to come from the blood (and humours) by way of food (e.g., Aristotle). With this in mind, "Avicenna's account is brief and clear: ingested food, having been transformed into chyle [lymph and emulsified fats] in the stomach, is subsequently transported to the liver and there concocted (literally, 'cooked') into blood, the two biles, and phlegm. Various stages of concoction purify the blood of superfluities which are excreted, and ultimately, part of the blood is refined into semen. Most of the blood, however, is used up in nourishing every part of the body. Hence, the parts of the body were said to be generated from the humours." See N. Siraisi, *Medieval ...*, p. 106. Cf. Aristotle, *De generatione animalium* [On the generation of animals]. Also see above *Coitus* and *Humours*.

Sensual: Used by Cornaro as a noun. Strictly speaking, both "sensist" or "sensationalist" are English terms more common to philosophical discourse from the seventeenth (e.g., Hobbes) and eighteenth centuries; as is the term "Sensualist" more common to the seventeenth century. In Cornaro's usage (following Plato, Galen, and others), the sensual, or that which is based on the appetites of the senses – is not a desirable trait in a man, since it fosters unrestrained and unchaste behaviour (*incontinenza*) that compromises his ability to reason. Cornaro's *sensuale* here is one who is overindulgent and animalistic.

Susan B. Mattern writes, "In general, Galen advocates a life of moderate sexuality and emphasizes the dangers of overindulgence more than those of restraint; in a culture where self-control, including sexual self-control, was a hallmark of masculinity, the athlete is once again an example of perverse extreme" (*Galen and the Rhetoric ...*, p. 130). Also see above, *Coitus*, and see *Sober ...*, p. 82n24.

Soul: Greek: *psuchē* (psyche); Latin: *anima*. *Oxford English Dictionary* defines this complex concept as: "The principle of thought and action in man, commonly regarded as an entity distinct from the body; the spiritual part of man in contrast to the purely physical. Also occas[ionally] the corresponding or analogous principle in animals. Freq[uently] in connexion with, or in contrast to, body. Sometimes personified, as in the common mediæval dialogues between the soul and the body ... 2a. The seat of the emotions, feelings or sentiments; the emotional part of man's nature ... 3b. Intellectual or spiritual power; high development of the mental faculties.... 6. Metaphysics, the vital sensitive or rational principle in plants, animals, or human beings ... 7b (fig. applied to persons) The personification of some quality ... 14a. Used with defining adjective, to denote a person of a particular character or in respect of some quality; frequently with a touch of contempt, compassion or familiarity" (*OED*, *s.v.*). In man, the soul "presides over all of his vegetative, sensitive and intellective functions" (Battaglia, *Grande Dizionario* ..., see *anima*, p. 478).

"Galen accepted the Platonic idea of the soul and distinguished three kinds: rational, choleric, and sensual (or rational, animal, and vegetative), residing in the brain, the heart, and liver, respectively. The rational soul governs reason, motion and sensation; the animal provides the 'vital force' of the body and is the source of emotions, the sensual, or vegetative, directs the process of nutrition and governs bodily needs. In other words, with the first one man thinks, the second is at the origin of his passions, and the third of his bodily desires" Plinio Prioreschi, *A History of Medicine: Roman Medicine* (Omaha, NE: Horatius Press, Vol. III, 1998, rpt 2001; p. 360). Also see below: *Spirit.*

Spirit: In Latin, *spiritus*. For the Stoics, it signifies the breath of God. The pneuma, in Greek, denotes *psuchē* (psyche: moth, butterfly) or soul, the vital conscious principle of every organism. "This idea of the spirit or pneuma which penetrates all the parts of the body was formulated in detail by the Stoics and developed by Galen [...] The breath or pneuma was thought to enter through the left side of the heart where it is converted into natural, vital and psychic force...then went to the brain whence it was distributed throughout the nervous system" (M. Ficino, *The Letters of Marsilio Ficino* ..., Vol. 2, p. 94, note 30:3). "Pneuma is above all the living form that permeates cosmic matter and determines the rational being" (Treccani, *Enciclopedia italiana, s.v.*). Animal spirit is seated in the brain (*pneuma physicon*, psychic faculty), the centre affecting the senses and movement; vital spirit, seated in the heart (*pneuma zoticon*, vital faculty), affects blood flow and temperature; natural spirit, seated in the liver (*pneuma physicon*, natural faculty), affects the nutrition and *metabolē* (metabolism) of the body. Any bad pneuma-spirit entering the body affects the various centres, the cause of *perturbatio*. Accidents of the soul or spirit include acts such as reasoning, striving, or worrying. Also see above: *Animo*, and *Soul.*

Taste: Here it refers to the pleasure of food for its flavour, or as the palate itself. Among the senses, taste has been philosophically ranked on either a lower order (e.g., Aristotle, *De anima*) or, as studied by Charles Burnett, on a higher one (anonymous, *Summa de saporibus*).

For further information on this thirteenth-century text, see Burnett, "The Superiority of Taste" in the *Journal of the Warburg and Courtauld Institutes* 54 (1991): pp. 230–8. On philosophy and taste, see for example, *Religion and the Senses in Early Modern Europe*, ed. Wietse de Boer and Christine Göttler (Leiden: Brill, 2013); or see, Carolyn Korsmeyer, *Making Sense of Taste: Food and Philosohy* (Ithaca, NY: Cornell University Press, 1999, 2002).

Temperament: Also known as *complexion*. It is associated with the four humours, and the four Empedoclean elements: air with the sanguine, water with the phlegmatic, fire with the choleric, and earth with the melancholic. According to Noga Arikha, "in turn, individual temperaments [*complexions*] were the product of variations in the proportion of each fluid in the body ... Women tended to be moist, old people dry ... Regardless of one's predominant temperament, however, humours shifted according to what one ate and drank, to where one lived, and to climate and season" (N. Arikha, *Passions ...*, p. xviii); "no doctor in his right mind would have diagnosed 'phlegmatic complexion' [for Giovanni de' Medici], just as no serious physician today believes that a good bleeding will reduce a temperature. Once the connection between disease and the existence of germs had been firmly established, about 150 years ago, it was indeed impossible to hold on to the theory of humours" (ibid.). Also see above: *Complexion, Elements,* and *Humours.*

Virtue: Italian, *virtù* (Greek, *aretē*). For Aristotle, *aretē* is "the activity of reason and rationally ordered habits" (*The Dictionary of Philosophy, s.v.,* 2001, p. 587), which are indicative of the virtues of intellect and the virtues of character (*The Cambridge Dictionary of Philosophy, s.v.,*1999, p. 43). It is also defined as a "force or energy, physical strength; the possession or display of manly [virile] qualities; manly excellence, manliness, courage, valour. Occult efficacy or power (as in the prevention or cure of disease, etc.), hence, a great worth or value. The efficacy arising from physical qualities; power to affect the human body in a beneficial manner; strengthening, sustaining, or healing properties" (*OED, s.v.*). It is the salubrious effect of food that is a virtue or power, for example, asparagus acts as a diuretic, and Ken Albala recounts that the eating of animal brains was thought to be good for the human intellect (K. Albala, *Eating Right ...,* p. 80).

Wine: The association of blood to wine that "seems to be an ancient one," is later evident in its use in the Holy Sacrament. Transubstantiation – drinking of the sacramental wine (or eating of the host-bread) that changes into the blood (or body) of Christ – was given an official definition for the Catholic Liturgy by the Council of Trent (1551).

"A dinner was called *prandium caninum vel abstemium,* at which no wine was drunk." This refers to "*quod canis vino caret* – because a dog drinks no wine" (Adam, Boyd, Da Ponte, *Roman Antiquities* ..., pp. 302nn5–6).

"Wine," moreover, "was considered an essential nutrient, in fact a meal without wine was called a *prandium caninum* or dog's dinner because only dogs have an aversion to wine. Wine was also drunk with breakfast, first thing in the morning" (K. Albala, *Food in Early Modern Europe* ..., p. 80).

Bibliography

Milani's Italian bibliography is not included here. Sources can be found in her notes to the "Introduction," or to her essay, "Immortality ...,". The reader can also refer to her Italian edition (*Scritti ...*, pp. 271-3).

Primary Sources

Cornaro, Alvise. *Alvise Cornaro: Scritti sulla vita sobria. Eulogio e Lettere.* La prima edizione critica a cura di Marisa Milani. Venezia: Corbo e Fiore Editori, 1983.
Milani, Marisa. "Come raggiungere l'immortalità vivendo cent'anni, ovvero La fortuna della 'Vita Sobria' nel mondo anglosassone." In *Cultura Neolatina,* nos. 4, 5, 6, vol. 40, pp. 333–56. Modena: S.T.E.M.- Mucchi, 1980.

Selected Bibliography

Adam, Alexander. *Roman Antiquities: Or an Account of the Manners and Customs of the Romans.* Additional notes by James Boyd and Lorenzo L. Da Ponte. New York: Collins, Keese & Co., 1837.
Albala, Ken. *Eating Right in the Renaissance.* Berkeley: University of California Press, 2002.
– *Food in Early Modern Europe.* Westport, CT: Greenwood Press, 2003.
– *The Banquet: Dining in the Great Courts of Renaissance Europe.* Urbana: University of Illinois Press, 2007.
Andrews, Richard. *Script and Scenarios: The Performance of Comedy in Renaissance Italy.* Cambridge: Cambridge University Press, 1993.

Arikha, Noga. *Passions and Tempers: A History of the Humours.* New York: Harper Collins, 2007.

Aurelius, Marcus. *Marcus Aurelius: Meditations.* Translated by A.S.L. Farquharson, introduction by D. A. Rees. New York: Random House, 1992.

Benham, W. Gurney. *A Book of Quotations, Proverbs and Household Words.* London: Cassell and Co. Ltd., 1907.

Brown, Horatio Robert Forbes. *Life on the Lagoons,* 5th ed. London: Rivingtons, 1909.

– "Marcantonio Bragadin, A Sixteenth-Century Cagliostro." In *Venetian Studies.* London: Elibron Classics Series, 2004. (Adamant Media Corporation's facsimile reprint of Kegan Paul, Trench & Co., London, 1887. Available at http://books.google.com. Accessed 6 May 2013.)

Bullough, Vern L. "Medieval Medical and Scientific Views of Women." In *Viator – Center for Medieval and Renaissance Studies,* vol. 4. Edited by Lynne White Jr., 485–501. Los Angeles: University of California Press, 1973.

Camporesi, Piero. *Bread of Dreams: Food and Fantasy in Early Modern Europe.* Translated by David Gentilcore. Cornwall, UK: Polity Press, T. J. Press (Padstow) Ltd., 1989.

– *Il Pane Selvaggio.* Bologna: Il Mulino, 1980.

Celenza, Christopher S. "The Revival of Platonic Philosophy." In *The Cambridge Companion to Renaissance Philosophy.* Edited by James Hankins. Cambridge: University of Cambridge Press, 2007.

Chiappini, Luciano. *La Corte estense alla metà del Cinquecento: i compendi di Cristoforo di Messisbugo.* Ferrara: Belriguardo, c1984.

Cornaro, Alvise. *Alvise Cornaro: La vita sobria.* A cura di Arnaldo Di Benedetto. Milano: TEA, 1993/1997.

– *Alvise Cornaro: Orazione per il Cardinale Marco Cornaro e Pianto per la morte del Bembo.* Due testi pavani inediti a cura di Marisa Milani. Bologna: Arti Grafiche Tamari, 1981.

Dante (Alighieri). *Dante: The Inferno.* Introduction and notes by Robert Hollander. Translated by Robert Hollander and Jean Hollander. New York: Doubleday, 2000.

– *The Divine Comedy of Dante Alighieri: Inferno.* Translated, introduction, and notes by Allen Mandelbaum. New York: Random House, Bantam Classic, 1982.

De Boer, Wietse, and Christine Göttler, eds. *Religion and the Senses in Early Modern Europe.* Leiden: Brill, 2013.

Diogenes (Laërtius). *Diogenes Laërtius: Lives of Eminent Philosophers,* vol. 2:X. Translated by Robert D. Hicks. Cambridge, MA: Harvard University Press, 1925/1995, p. 655 and p. 657.

di Schino, June, and Furio Luccichenti. *Il cuoco segreto dei papi. Bartolomeo Scappi e la Confraternita dei cuochi e dei pasticcieri.* Roma: Gangemi Editore, 2007.

Farrar, Frederic W. *Lives of the Fathers: Sketches of Church History in Biography.* New York: MacMillan, 1889.

Ficino, Marsilio. *The Letters of Marsilio Ficino.* Translated by the Language Department of the School of Economic Science, London. Vol. 2, Liber III. London: Fellowship of the School of Economic Science, London-Shepheard-Walwyn, 1978.

– *Three Books on Life.* Critical edition, translation and notes by Carol V. Kaske and John R. Clark. Binghampton, NY: Medieval & Renaissance Texts and Studies in conjunction with the Renaissance Society of America, 1989.

Frascari, Marco. "Honestamente Bella, Alvise Cornaro's Temperate View of Lady Architecture and Her Maids, Phronesis and Sophrosine." McGill University lecture, 2007. First posted online 17 March 2008. Available at http://www.arch.mcgill.ca/theory/conference/papers/Frascari_Cornaro.pdf. Accessed 6 May 2013.

Gullino, Giuseppe. "Corner, Alvise." In *Dizionario Biografico degli Italiani,* vol. 29. Istituto della Enciclopedia Italiana Fondata da Giovanni Treccani. Roma: Società Grafica Romana, 1983.

Harrison, Peter. "Philosophy and the Crisis of Religion." In *The Cambridge Companion to Renaissance Philosophy.* Edited by James Hankins. Cambridge: University of Cambridge Press, 2007.

Jütte, Robert. *Poverty and Deviance in Early Modern Europe.* Cambridge: Cambridge University Press, 2001 (first printed 1994, reprint 1996, 1999).

Lippi, Emilio. *Cornariana: Studi su Alvise Cornaro.* Padova: Bliblioteca Veneta I: Editrice Antenore, 1983.

Longrigg, James. *Greek Rational Medicine: Philosophy and Medicine from Alcmaeon to the Alexandrians.* London-NYC: Routledge, 1993.

Mattern, Susan B. *Galen and the Rhetoric of Healing.* Baltimore: The Johns Hopkins University Press, 2008.

Mazzotta, Giuseppe. *Cosmopoiesis: The Renaissance Experiment.* Toronto: University of Toronto Press, 2001.

Menegazzo, Emilio. "Altre osservazioni intorno alla vita e all'ambiente del Ruzante e del Alvise Cornaro." In *Italia Medioevale e Umanistica,* vol. 9. Padova: Editrice Antenore, 1966.

Muir, Edward. *The Culture Wars of the Late Renaissance: Skeptics, Libertines, and Opera.* The Bernard Berenson Lectures on the Italian Renaissance sponsored by Villa I Tatti. Cambridge, MA: Harvard University Press, 2007.

Proctor, Robert E. *Defining the Humanities: How Rediscovering a Tradition Can Improve Our Schools.* Bloomington: Indiana University Press, 1988, 1998.

Puppi, Lionello, ed. *Alvise Cornaro e il suo tempo.* Catalogo della mostra a cura di Lionello Puppi. Comune di Padova, Assessorato ai beni cuturali. Loggio e Odeo Cornaro. Sala del Palazzo della Regione, 7 Settembre–9 Novembre 1980.

Sambin, Paolo. *Per le biografie di Angelo Beolco, il Ruzante, e di Alvise Cornaro, Rivisti e aggiornati da Francesco Padovan.* Padova: Esedra Editrice, 2002.

Sanudo, Marin (Marin Sanuto). *Itinerario di Marin Sanuto per la terraferma veneziana nell'anno MCCCCLXXXIII.* Padua: Tipografia del seminario, 1847. Available at http://books.google.com. Accessed 7 May 2013.

Scappi, Bartolomeo. *The* Opera *of Bartolomeo Scappi. L'arte et prudenza d'un maestro cuoco. The Art and Craft of a Master Cook.* Translated with commentary by Terence Scully. Lorenzo Da Ponte Italian Library. Toronto: University of Toronto Press, 2008.

Siraisi, Nancy G. *The Clock and the Mirror: Girolamo Cardano and Renaissance Medicine.* Princeton, NJ: Princeton University Press, 1997.

– *Medieval and Early Renaissance Medicine: An Introduction to Knowledge and Practice.* Chicago: University of Chicago Press, 1990.

Speroni, Sperone. *Sperone Speroni, Lettere familiari.* Tomo secondo Lettere a diversi. A cura di Maria Rosa Loi e Mario Pozzi. Alessandria: Edizioni dell'Orso s.a.s., 1994.

Squatriti, Paolo. *Water and Society in Early Medieval Italy AD 400–1000.* Cambridge: Cambridge University Press, 1998.

Tafuri, Manfredo. *Venezia e il Rinascimento.* Torino: Giulio Einaudi, 1985.

– *Venice and the Renaissance.* Translated by Jessica Levine. Cambridge, MA: MIT Press, 1995.

Tripp, Edward. *Crowell's Handbook of Classical Mythology.* Edited by Edward Tripp. New York: Harper Collins, 1970.

Virgil. *The Aeneid of Virgil.* Edited and an introduction by T.E. Page. London-Toronto: St. Martin's Press-MacMillan, 1894/1962.

Wilkes, K.V. "Psuchē versus Mind." In *Essays on Aristotle's De Anima.* Edited by Martha C. Nussbaum and Amélie Oksenberg Rorty. Oxford: Oxford University Press, 1988/1998.

Zanré, Domenico. *Cultural Non-Conformity in Early Modern Florence.* Aldershot, UK: Ashgate, 2004.

Reference Works

Abbagnano, Nicola, ed. *Dizionario di filosofia.* Torino: UTET, 1961; reprint and revised 1968.

Audi, Robert, ed. *The Cambridge Dictionary of Philosophy.* Cambridge: Cambridge University Press, 1995/2001.

Battaglia, Salvatore. *Grande dizionario della lingua italiana.* Edited by Bárberi Squarotti. Turin: UTET, 1961–2002.

Florio, John. *John Florio's Worlde of Wordes.* Critical edition and edited by
  Hermann Haller. Lorenzo Da Ponte Italian Library. Toronto: University of
  Toronto Press, 2013; first printed London, 1598.
Oxford English Dictionary, Compact Disc. 2nd ed. Oxford: Oxford University Press,
  1992.
Runes, Dagobert D., ed. *The Dictionary of Philosophy.* New York: Citadel Press,
  2001.
Treccani, Giovanni. *Enciclopedia italiana di scienze, lettere ed arti.* Pubblicata sotto
  l'alto patronato di S.M. il Re d'Italia. Roma: Istituto dell'Enciclopedia Itali-
  ana fondata da Giovanni Treccani, 1925–2006.
– *Dizionario Biografico degli Italiani.* Istituto della Enciclopedia Italiana Fondata
  da Giovanni Treccani. Roma: Società Grafica Romana, 1983.

Index

defined, 61n**; lexicon, 3n**; poetry, 63; the *Ruzanti* and, 61
Pavano Academy, 62, 63, 63n110
Pellico, Silvio, 38
Percacino (or Percachino), Grazioso, 3, 8, 8n12, 12, 15, 17, 62n108, 184
perturbations, 113; Cornaro and, 94, 96, 105; humours, 21; illness and, 21; reason and, 127, 165, 176; soul and, 19; terminology, xxvii, 218; types of, 28, 83, 164; vice and, 92, 172
Peru, 38
pestilence, 9, 9n14, 52; banquets as, 77, 78; Tomitano and, 74n5
Petrarch (Petrarca), Francesco, 94n41
Petrinella (Petrinella da Armer di Candia), 65, 66, 66n111, 67; daughter of, 136n10
Petrobelli, Maria Paola: on the Odeo, 39, 39n64
Petrucci, Franceschina: Cornaro creditor, 58
Philodemus, 170n44
Philo. *See* Judaeus of Alexandria, Philo
philosophers, 24, 188, 216, 217; Alcmaeon, 76n9; on animo, 214; Cornaro and, 19, 24, 117, 174, 180; Speroni on 143, 147, 152; Tomitano, 8, 74
phlegm (*flemma*), 20, 21n35, 87n31, 216, 217, 219, 221
Phoebus, 30, 131, 132n2
physician: alchemy and, 30; amused by, 119; Cornaro versus, 10, 19, 24, 86, 160, 207; diet and, 25, 26n41; limitation of, 10; one's own, 87, 88, 200; perfect, 25, 87, 88; in poetry, 63, 63n*; prescriptions by, 29, 31, 119; radical moisture and, 79n17;

role of, 88; and the sober life, 14, 87, 88, 199, 207; in Speroni, 140; temperament and, 221
Piccolomini, Alessandro, 60
pill, 30, 118
Pino, Paolo, 14, 33n54, 170n46
Pisani, Francesco di Alvise, 54, 58, 65, 117n64, 157n33, 186
Pitti Palace: Cornaro portrait by Tintoretto, 206, 206n*
Pius IV, Aretino and, 111n58; 146n10
plagiarism, 38
plagiarizes, 32n51
plague, 8; Asclepius and, 140n2; Bembo and, 154; Bubonic, 77n12
Plato, 90n35, 122, 143n6, 179n53, 180, 189, 215, 219; dietary norms, 76n9; elements and, 87n31; order and, 89, 90; *Republic*, 174; and the soul, 220
Platonism, 170n44
play, 46; comic, 46, 47n80, 133; in poetry, 62; Sophocles, 97n43
pleasure, 212; Cornaro's, 94–6, 113, 118, 119, 124, 127, 135, 156, 176–7; Epicureanism and, 169nn44–5; Ethics and, 105n52; gluttony and, 104; pain and, 170n45; soul and, 92; of taste, 78, 78n14, 116, 170n45, 220
poetry, 59; patron of, 135; Pavano, 61n**
Poland, 38
polemic: with physicians, 10; with Speroni, 186
poor, the: *boari* as, 62; bread and, 52n92, 215; Cornaro and, 29, 53, 68, 114, 115, 115n63; diet of, 28, 29; disparity among, 29, 53n*; sober life and, 29, 100